Data Collection And Analysis

How to Take, Read and Interpret Radiographs for the Prognosis and Treatment of the Foundered Horse

by

Dr. Esco Buff

Dear Steve,
Thanks for your support and being great customers,
Esco
6/05

Library of Congress Control Number: 2005901430

ISBN: 0-9766350-0-3

First printing March 2005

Additional copies of this book are available by mail.
For more information or ordering contact:

Esco Buff, PhD, CF
Esco Buff's Farrier and Founder Service
1347 Robin Hood Lane
Webster, New York 14580
(585) 298-6619
www.escobuff.com

Printed in the U.S.A. by
Morris Publishing
3212 East Highway 30
Kearney, NE 68847
800-650-7888

DEDICATION

This book is dedicated to
my wife Christine Buff,
our children,
Jeremy, Victoria, Alec and Cory;
To all my Family and Friends;
To my mentor and friend,
Doug Butler;
And most of all to our Heavenly Father
for showing me the way.

ACKNOWLEDGMENTS

The author is indebted to many people who have encouraged and suggested the need for a more in depth publication that would help explain how to fully use and understand the
Founder Data Collection and Analysis Form ©.

I want to especially acknowledge the following individuals for their help and support, without which this book would never have come to light.

Christine Buff, my soul mate and partner in life. To put up with my unbridled spirit, frustrations and joys. Thank you for your support, feedback and love. It was Christine, knowing my strong interest in foundered horses, who first suggested to me, *"Why don't you write a book?"*

Doug Butler, PhD, CJF, FWCF, for your tremendous leadership in the Farrier profession, your friendship, and for being a powerful influence and mentor.
Thank you for your encouragement, feedback and support. I offer a heartfelt thank you.

Robert Eustace, BVSc, Cert E.O., Cert E.P., FRCVS, for your friendship, wisdom and guidance. Thank you for your dedication to laminitic and foundered horse.

King Lamadora, for your friendship, encouragement and support. It is now my turn to encourage you to write a book on Limb Length Disparities and Proper Balance Movement (PBM II).

Mark Flaherty, for your friendship, support, farrier assistance, and ability to provide excellent feedback and constructive criticism.

Rolfe M. Radcliffe, DVM, DACVS, for your friendship and professional guidance with the making and editing of this book.

Jennifer A. Reetz, DVM, Dip ACVIM, for being kind enough to write the foreword and for your professional guidance, feedback and continual commitment to the horse and horse owner.

David K. Trachtenberg, DVM and the
Staff of Ledgewood Equine Veterinary Clinic, PC,
for your support, patience and commitment, radiographing the many foundered horse that come into the clinic.

I also acknowledge the help, support and suggestions of many veterinarians, farriers and horse owners.

Writing this book has truly been a joy.

Esco Buff, PhD, CF

About the Author

Esco Buff, PhD, CF is the owner of Esco Buff's Farrier and Founder Service. He is an American Farriers Association Certified Farrier with 30 years experience trimming and shoeing horses.

Esco Resides in Upstate New York with his wife, Christine and their four children, Jeremy, Victoria, Alec and Cory.

Mr.. Buff is a graduate of New Mexico State Farrier School under Mogens I. Rasmussen or "Rass" and the Illinois State Horseshoeing School. He hold a Bachelor of Science in Psychology, a Masters in Science, and a Doctorate of Philosophy in Business Administration.

Esco Buff is dedicated to excellence in horse foot care. He has a strong interest in working with foundered and limb length disparity horses. Through applying the principles of hoof balance and biomechanics, Esco Buff creates sound horses with healthy functioning feet.

Dr. Esco Buff is a recognized leader in the field of founder farrier treatment and is routinely consulted for horse's that are foundered or with therapeutic shoeing needs. He typically shoes between 60 to 70 new-foundered horse cases per year.

In the past twelve years (1991 to 2003), Esco has documented and shod over 625 new-foundered cases with a 98% survival rate. Of these, 83% returned to their original state of soundness, 16% were unable to return to their original state of soundness and 2% were euthanized.

Due to his extensive experience in shoeing foundered horses, Dr. Buff designed and published, ***The Founder Data Collection and Analysis Form ©.***

The forms are clear, concise and easy to use. The forms and instruction sheet teach consistent radiograph techniques, thus enabling the veterinarian and farrier to obtain more accurate information in order to assess, determine prognosis and establish treatment for the foundered horse.

Esco shares his knowledge with an enthusiasm and dedication that reflects his love for the horse and his trade. His knowledge of the farrier craft makes him a natural for consultations, group teaching experiences and as a presenter at workshop, seminars and clinics.

Dr. Buff is an international speaker who has presented on many topics including: Foundered Horseshoeing, Limb Length Disparities, The Principles of Balance, How to Set up and Run a Successful Farrier Business, Farrier Business Skills, Preventive Foot Care, Hoof Wall Repairs and Resections, Effective Communication, and Lameness Problem Solving.

Foreword

New information about the etiologies and pathogenesis of laminitis and founder has emerged since I graduated veterinary school.

Over that same period, numerous new preventative measures and treatment have also appeared. It is commonly felt that the more treatments there are for a disease process, the lower the probability of one treatment being more successful than another. This statement is quite applicable to laminitis and founder.

However, after meeting and working with Dr. Esco Buff on numerous laminitis and founder cases, my feelings regarding treatment, as well as assessing prognosis, have changed. I have been amazed at the success of various cases from the acutely foundered horse to the cases of sinkers and chronic type II's.

Numerous clients of mine were thrilled with the outcome of their foundered horse, and were very appreciative of my involving Dr. Esco Buff to aid in the immediate and long-term treatment.

I now believe that it is crucial to involve an experienced farrier at the onset of foundered cases, in addition to working with the farrier through the subsequent days, weeks and months.

I'm convinced of the higher probability of success when using **properly placed heart bar shoes** in pre-acute, acute and chronic cases, along with identifying and treating any underlying causes.

The Founder Data Collection and Analysis Form ©, has given veterinarians and farriers a better method for assessing the severity of laminitis and founder, and provides a more accurate prognosis and monitoring of a horse's progress over time.

I thank Dr. Esco Buff for teaching me a new adjunctive method to approach cases of laminitis and found. I know the clients and the horses thank him too.

Jennifer A. Reetz, DVM, Dip. ACVIM

Contents

Introduction

There are several theories attempting to explain the mechanisms of laminitis and founder. It is not the goal of this book to delve into these theories. **The goal of this book** is to provide the veterinarian, farrier and horse owner with **the most successful** treatment techniques now that the horse has foundered.

It is wise to treat and shoe the horse with the principles, techniques and tools that will provide the highest chance of success. These principles and techniques should be based on the **understanding of** the foot's biomechanics and circulatory system.

Unfortunately, out-dated treatment and unconventional or unorthodox shoeing techniques, which go against the above, are still being applied. Many of these treatment actually worsen the founder condition and confronting these techniques can be frustrating for the educated professional.

As Uk's **Simon Curtis, FWCF, Hon. Assoc. RCVS** has stated, *"It is hard to confront a simple lie with a complex truth."*

Some veterinarians and farriers will tend to look at each horse individually, using different treatments, trimming and shoeing techniques. The author has seen much higher success rates by developing a more defined approach that works in a majority of foundered horse; then, as needed, adapted to fit each individual horse.

So what is laminitis and founder?

Laminitis is a reduction of blood flow to the laminae secondary to inflammation. If the blood supply is interrupted for only a short time, little to no permanent damage results. The more severe and longer the reduction in blood supply, the greater the chances of irreversible damage. Once the reduction of blood supply caused failure in the laminae between the distal phalanx and hoof capsule, the animal is considered foundered.

Founder is a complicated systemic disease resulting from a triggering insult. In order to provide the highest chances of success, the horse is best served through the **collaboration** of a qualified veterinarian and farrier.

General practitioner farriers should not attempt to shoe foundered horses, but rather refer them to an experienced farrier.

Doug Butler, PhD, CJF, FWCF, writes, *"Any farrier or veterinarian who decides to tackle founder alone, without the cooperation of the other, does not have the best interest of the animal nor of the owner in mind."*

The veterinarian's role is to diagnosis the insult, if at all possible, and provide treatment for the triggering insult and any systemic problems. They will also provide radiographs for the prognosis, treatment and monitoring of the horse.

The farrier's role is to provide mechanical and bone column support via the heart bar shoe.

This book will provide information important before, during and after treatment of a foundered horse. It is intended to relay the most successful treatment approach based on the author's and others experiences.

Although the author has shod many foundered horses, ponies, minature ponies/horses, donkeys, minature donkeys and mules, this method of radiograph analysis **can only be applied** to the horse and pony. Donkeys and Mules have slightly different foot anatomy, even though the techniques for applying a heart bar shoe are the same.

Currently, the author is in the process of establishing methods to help determine prognosis and guidelines for the treatment of the foundered mule or donkey.

Chapter One will cover techniques to provide more comfort for the horse, until veterinarian and farrier treatment can be provided.

Chapter Two will discuss specific radiograph techniques in order to provide data necessary for the assessment, prognosis, and treatment of the foundered horse.

Chapter Three will teach you how to collect and document data taken from the radiograph with the aid of **The Founder Data Collection and Analysis Form ©.**

Chapter Four will cover how to use the data collected to make a determination on the prognosis for survival and the chances the horse will return to its useful soundness state.

Chapter Five will cover how to use the radiographs to shoe the horse with rigid heart bar shoes.

Chapter Six will provide a summary and discuss aftercare instructions in order to maximize treatment success.

Laminitis and Founder is a complex disease with significant animal, human and economic impacts. The cases are often frustrating and clinically challenging to manage.

The most significant consequence of founder is that it remains a potentially crippling performance limiting, life threatening disease.

Over the years, many people have proposed many devices and methods that they claim are cure-alls. No one device or method works 100% of the time, but some work with a higher percentage than others.

Such a method **does not compromise the blood supply** to the already damaged laminae of the foot. The heart bar shoe fits this protocol.

This book is based on such methods and will help instill in the reader sound principles to provide the highest chances of success.

Chapter 1

Emergency First Aid

before treatment begins

First and foremost, you will need to get immediate treatment started by calling in a qualified **veterinarian and farrier.** Early treatment is crucial to minimize the damage incurred and increase the chances of success.

Other than support limb laminitis/founder, laminitis/founder really does occur in all four feet. Some will say they have seen it in the front, not in the hind, in one foot, and not the others. Upon closer examination, you will find that all four feet do undergo some laminae stress, distortion or even separation. However, it may be that all four feet get different treatments. Most horses do not require hind frog support shoes.

If the horse is shod, **do not** pull the shoes as they are providing some support. The only reason to remove the shoes is if the current shoe is causing more harm than good, to fit a correctly placed heart bar shoe or at the time the veterinarian takes the radiographs.

Do not fit any device that could or will apply pressure to the sole of the foot, such as Styrofoam ™, sole packing, sole pressure shoes, full pads, etc.

The sole **is not** designed as a weight bearing structure. Devices that apply sole pressure can cause abscesses, bruising, destroy the blood supply and **do not** provide support to the bone column.

It is the author's opinion that anyone, especially veterinarians and farriers, that apply Styrofoam ™, sole packing or any other type of sole pressure/contact items, are admitting how little they understand about founder and the vascular anatomy of the foot.

A correctly fitted frog support system will improve the comfort for most laminitic and foundered horses. The horses gain immediate relief and alter their stance to a more normal position. There are several types of frog support systems that can be used, however, the author has seen improved results with the application of rolled gauze or 4x4 bandages.

The principle of fitting frog supports is to increase the thickness of the horse's frog so that during weight bearing, some of the forces are transferred through the frog. This helps decrease the forces acting through the wall, thus reducing the strain on already damaged laminae.

The frog should be tested before fitting frog supports. This can be done by using hoof testers or your thumbs to apply pressure to all parts of the frog. Sore frogs may result from previous excessive frog supports or from seromas (fluid accumulation) beneath the frog and sole.

If the horse is **positive to frog pressure** and overly sensitive on the frogs, do not fit frog supports. Leave the horse in a deeply bedded stall until the veterinarian and farrier have assessed the horse.

Using rolled gauze or 4x4 gauze pads can provide a temporary frog support first-aid measure. Fitting frog supports is much easier with two people, but can be accomplished with one person. One person can hold up the foot and the other can do the bandaging.

First, pick up the foot and clean it out thoroughly of debris. If you're the farrier or veterinarian, trim the frog so there will be equal support. The horse owner should fit the frog support system to an untrimmed frog.

Whichever bandage material you use, place them directly on the frog for constant support. Place the bandage one-half (½") back from the apex or point of frog (figure 1.1).

Adjust the bandage so it is about one-half inch (½") higher than the hoof wall at the heels. The bandage material should compress down enough so there is equal weight bearing on the frog and hoof wall. This can be tested before you finish bandaging by placing a stiff straight piece of wood or metal across the heels and pushing down with your thumbs (figure 1.2). Remove or add bandage material until you have equal contact of the frog and hoof wall.

Now tape them into position with elastic bandage or similar bandage material. Be sure not to bandage tightly over the coronary band and the heel bulbs (figure 1.3).

Return the horse to a deeply bedded stall.

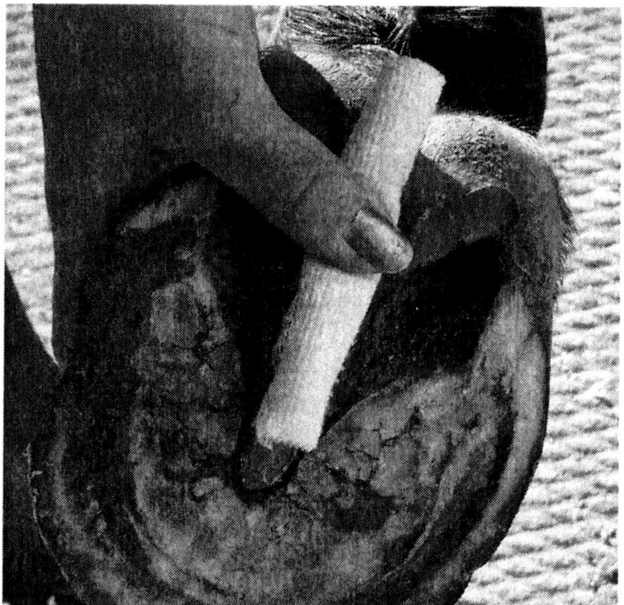

Figure 1.1 - Fitting a frog support made of folded over 4x4's.

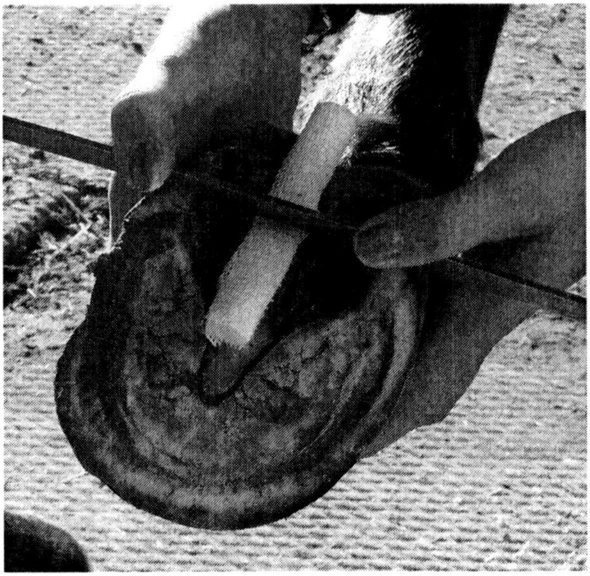

Figure 1.2 - Compression of bandage material showing correct thickness when pressure is applied.

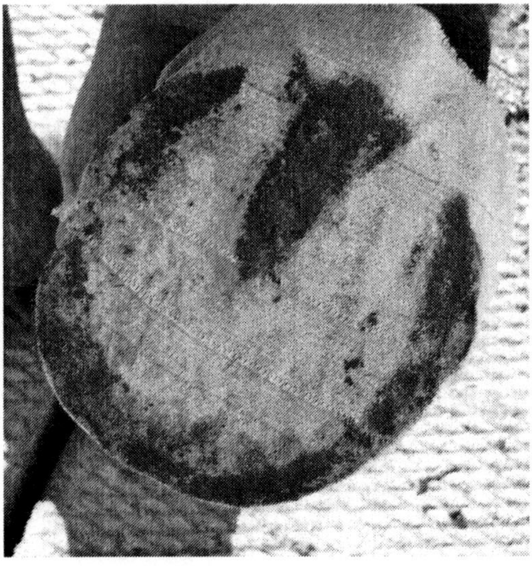

Figure 1.3 - Frog support in place, bandaged and showing weight bearing on frog and hoof wall only.

Until seen by the veterinarian and farrier, stable the horse in at least ten to twelve inches of clean, dry shavings. Such bedding allows the lying horse to more comfortable and the standing horse to set its heels into the shavings at whatever height it finds most comfortable. Horses do this by pushing the toe down into the shavings and/or by mounding up piles of shavings to place their heels and frogs onto.

With the horse now in a deeply bedded stall and the frog support system applied, the horse will now have a greater chance of minimizing further laminar damage, until the veterinarian and farrier can provide further treatment.

Remember, early and correct treatment is crucial to minimize the damage incurred and increase the chances of success.

Chapter 2

Radiograph Techniques

to help aid in the assessment and prognosis of the foundered horse

A few **simple preliminaries** will make the difference between a radiograph that is useful for diagnostic and prognostic purposes and one that is not.

Two wooden blocks are needed about 2 ½" to 3" high and wide enough for the horse to stand on. Lateromedial views of the distal phalanx normally require the foot to be raised of sufficient thickness to bring the solar surface of the foot level with the center of the radiograph beam. This also allows the bottom of the cassette to be placed lower than the solar surface of the foot so that it is included on the film.

A cut off bicycle spoke or metal rod is embedded into the top of the wooden block to highlight the ground surface.

Preparation of the horse **is essential** to good radiographs. Quiet horses will reduce movement. The horse's foot should be brushed/cleaned out and the frog and sole should have any defoliation removed. A clean foot will help eliminate confusing artifacts.

The frog does not show up well on lateromedial radiographs. In order to show the frog in relation to the distal phalanx, a tack is used to highlight the apex of the frog.

The tack is merely a reference point to determine proper placement of the toe and frog plate on the heart bar shoe. The tack is pushed into the apex of the frog. **The exact placement is not as important as long** as its position on the frog is marked in some way. A heavy felt tip pen is ideal for marking the frog and sole (figure 2.1).

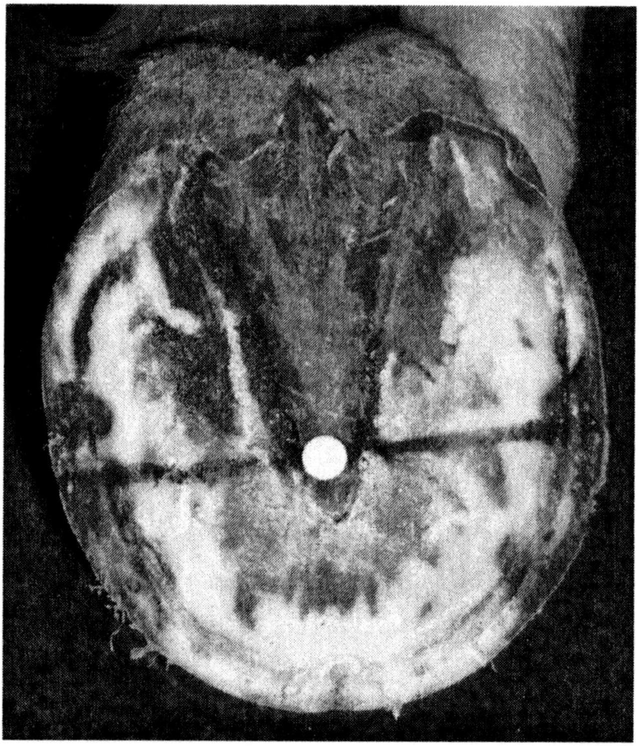

Figure 2.1 - Solar view of the foot showing tack placement and marker line.

For **prognostic purposes**, another marker is used on the front of the hoof wall. A straight stiff wire of known length (about 50 to 60 mm) is used to highlight the front and top of the hoof wall. A piece of copper or steel wire works best. **Do Not** use flexible or braided wire as this makes radiographic interpretation more difficult.

The length of the wire must be known so the effects of radiographic magnification can be adjusted.

The wire is taped to the hoof wall so the top of the wire is located where the wall changes from hard to soft (figure 2.2). In Chapter 4 we will explain how the position of the wire will aid in determining the prognosis of survival and return soundness.

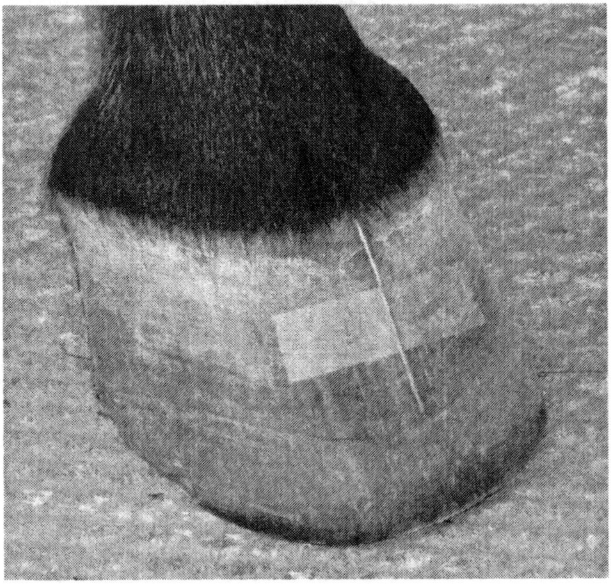

Figure 2.2 - View of the foot showing placement of the dorsal wall wire marker.

The horse should stand with one foot on each block with the cannon bone vertical (figure 2.3). This is the ideal situation, however many of us deal with horse's that can't even stand.

In a well-positioned radiograph, the radiograph beam is perpendicular to the cassette to avoid image distortion. The radiograph beam should be parallel to the top of the block and perpendicular to the axis of the limb so that precise lateromedial radiographs are produced. The importance of a true lateromedial radiograph cannot be overemphasized for proper interpretation.

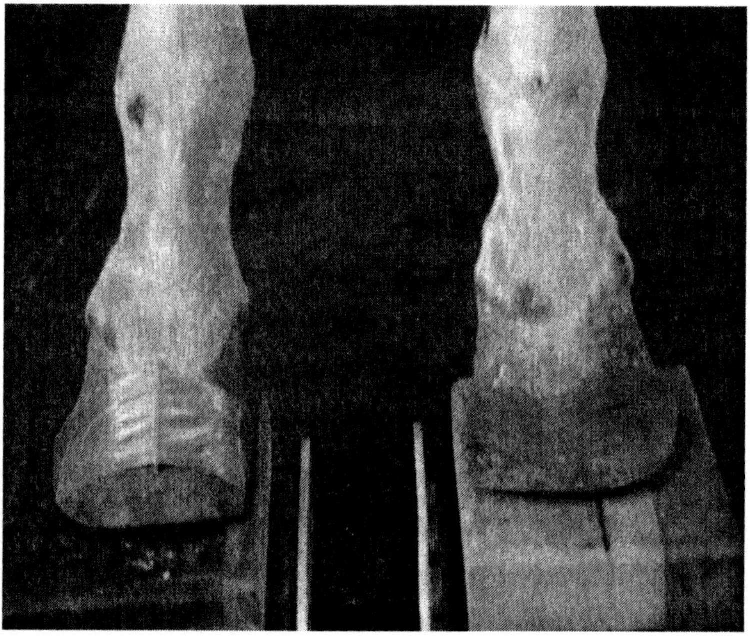

Figure 2.3 - A foundered horse ready for radiographing.

Chapter 3

How to Collect and Document Data from the Radiographs

with the aid of the Founder Data Collection and Analysis Form (FDCAA) ©

Once the radiograph has been developed, you are now ready to collect the data. **Consistency** and **double-checking** is recommended. Measure twice, cut once.

Before collecting the data, the author suggests placing a clear sheet of plastic, report cover, etc. over the radiograph, in order to avoid leaving marks that could interfere with current and future radiograph analysis. Another method is to use a colored China Marker ™ on the radiographs, which can be easily wiped off without damaging the radiograph.

The Founder Data Collection and Analysis Form © (figure 3.1) will aid in the collection of data.

The forms are clear and concise and include a laminated instruction sheet that enables the veterinarian and farrier to more accurately assess, determine prognosis and establish treatment for the foundered horse.

The forms along with this book will help the professional determine the chances that the horse will return to its previous soundness state. The forms teach consistent radiograph techniques, thus enabling the veterinarian and farrier to obtain more accurate information from the radiographs. They also help determine where to correctly place the frog plate of the heart bar shoe.

Doug Butler, PhD, CJF, FWCF has written, *"Esco has developed a form than can help veterinarians and farriers in three ways:*

1. *Establish a common language of visualization for farrier and veterinarian communication to help them predict probable outcome.*

2. *Help teach horse owners the seriousness of their horse's condition and help them make treatment decisions.*

3. *Document change when treatment is not effective and/or gives needed protection in the event of litigation.*

I recommend the method of mechanical treatment and documentation he has detailed in these forms."

The Founder Data Collection and Analysis Forms © are three part, carbonless, 8 ½" x 11" data sheets, sold in sets of 25 per package. Each set includes a laminated Instruction Sheet, which contains detailed instructions discussing radiograph techniques, how to interpret the radiographic measurements, how to correct for magnification, and how to analyze the data in order to apply a correct frog plate and hear bar shoe.

These forms can be obtained by contacting the author or through several farrier supply stores.

The data to be collected (figure 3.2) from the radiograph will be:

- Actual length of wire
- Radiographic length of wire
- Wall thickness (WT)
- Founder distance (D)
- Founder Type
- Frog plate placement calculation (F)
- Shoe toe placement calculation (ST)
- P-3 (distal phalanx) angle (Angle T)
- Dorsal wall angle (Angle T)
- Phalanx angle (Angle S)
- Palmar cortex of the phalanx length (L)

FOUNDER DATA COLLECTION AND ANALYSIS FORM

Owner ______________________

Veterinarian ______________________

Farrier ______________________

Horse ______________________

Breed ______________________

Gender __________ Age __________

Date of Radiograph ______________________

Date of Data Collection ______________________

Front Hind

Left Right

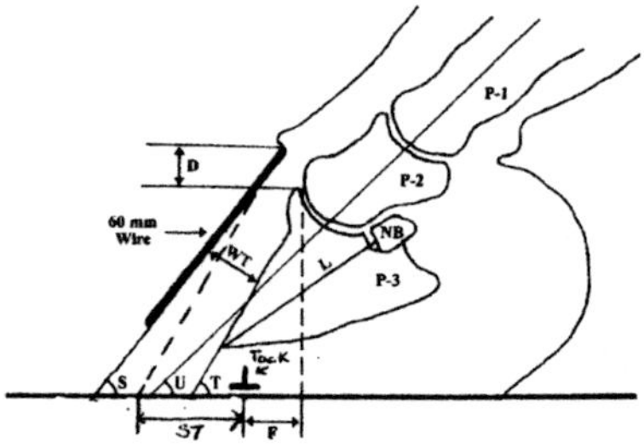

Wire Length

Actual = ______________ mm

Radiologically = ______________ mm

Founder Type

Laminitis Acute CT-I CT-II Sinker

Magnification Correction = Length Measured Radiographically X Actual Wire Length / Radiographic Wire Length

= ______________ mm

= ______________ mm

Angle S (Dorsal Wall Angle) = __________ degrees

Angle T (P-3 Angle) = __________ degrees

Angle U (Phalanx Angle) = __________ degrees

Angle of Hoof Capsule Rotation = Angle T (______) **minus** Angle S (______) = __________ degrees
Angle of Distal Phalanx Rotation = Angle T (______) **minus** Angle U (______) = __________ degrees

L (Palmer Cortex of the Distal Phalanx Distance)

Radiologically = ______________ mm

Corrected for Magnification = ______________ mm

F (Frog Plate Placement Calculation)

Radiologically = ______________ mm

Corrected for Magnification = ______________ mm

WT (Wall Thickness)

Radiologically = ______________ mm

Corrected for Magnification = ______________ mm

Normal Wall Thickness (L x .25) = ______________ mm

ST (Shoe Toe Placement Calculation)

Radiologically = ______________ mm

Corrected for Magnification = ______________ mm

D (Founder Distance)

Radiologically = ______________ mm

Corrected for Magnification = ______________ mm

Veterinarian/Farrier Treatment to Date and Any Other Concurrent Problems:
(Abscess, Serum Pockets, Infectious Osteitis, Pedal Osteitis, Osteomyelitis, Dropped Sole, Prolapsed Sole, Ringbone, Sidebones....)

____

____

Figure 3.1 - A blank Founder Data Collection and Analysis Form ©.

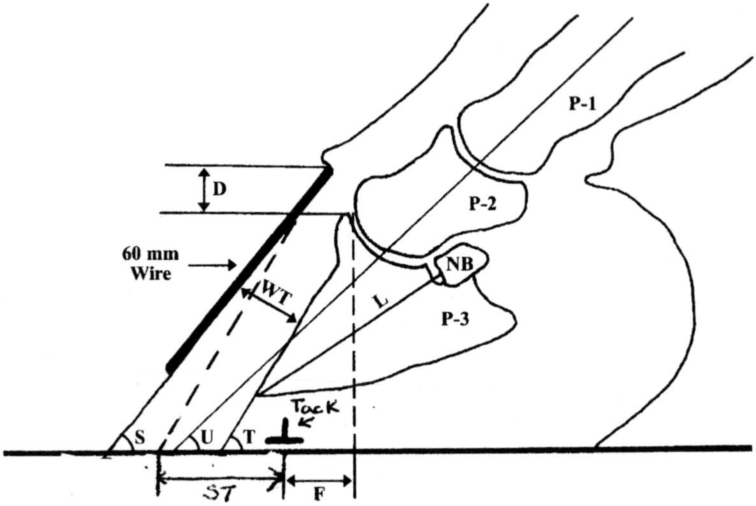

Figure 3.2 - Data to be collected from The Founder Data Collection and Analysis Form ©.

Actual and Radiographic Wire Length

The actual wire length is the actual length of the dorsal wall wire marker used. The radiographic wire length is the measured length of the dorsal wall wire marker from the radiograph.

These two measurements will be needed so the effects of radiographic magnification can be adjusted for correct interpretation of the radiograph.

It is of the **utmost importance** to know the actual length of the wire so the farrier can correctly and precisely fit the frog plate of the heart bar shoe. **Arbitrarily using** an unknown wire length to mark the dorsal hoof wall will prevent the farrier from being able to apply the heart bar **shoe correctly.**

Magnification Correction

In order to get actual working measurements, calculations need to be made in order to correct for the radiographic magnification.

This calculation is important in order to be able to assess prognosis, remove the correct amount of dorsal hoof wall and to correctly place your frog plate on the heart bar shoe.

The magnification formula is:

$$\frac{\text{actual wire length}}{\text{radiographic wire length}} \times \text{length measured Radiographically that you are looking to correct}$$

Example:

A 60 mm wire was used. Radiographic length of wire was 68 mm. Using the formula:

60 divided by 68 equals 0.8823529 mm or 0.88 mm
60/68 = 0.8823529 mm = 0.88 mm

Wall Thickness (WT) (figure 3.2)

Wall thickness is the distance from the wire marker on the dorsal hoof wall to the dorsal cortex of the distal phalanx. This is measured half way up dorsally from the tip of the distal phalanx to the base of the extensor process, and at a right angle to the dorsal cortex of the distal phalanx.

Wall thickness, uncorrected for magnification, **greater than 13-15 mm for miniatures, 15-17 mm for horses and 17-19 mm for drafts**, is an indicator that they may be foundering and laminar separation has occurred.

This point is very important and quite often overlooked by many veterinarians and farriers.

In the early stages of founder, the hoof wall and the distal phalanx will draw apart an move downward, but remain parallel. Rotation of the distal phalanx occurs later. By recognizing these early signs, the veterinarian and farrier can provide immediate treatment that could help limit the amount of damage sustained.

Palmar Cortex of the Distal Phalanx Length (L) (figure 3.2)

This is the length of the palmar cortex of the distal phalanx from the tip of the distal phalanx to the articulation of the distal phalanx and the navicular bone.

The length of the palmar cortex of the distal phalanx can be used as an assessment tool in order to see how much, if any, of the distal phalanx has remodeled.

Christopher Pollitt, BVSc, PhD, has shown that the wall thickness in the normal horse is approximately 25% of L (corrected for magnification). Wall thickness greater than this, is an indicator that the horse may be foundering. The normal wall thickness calculation can also be used to help determine how much dorsal hoof wall needs to be removed.

Founder Distance (D) (figure 3.2)

Founder distance is the vertical distance between the top of the dorsal hoof wall marker and the proximal limit of the extensor process of the distal phalanx.

Founder distance **is the most useful radiological prognostic indicator** for acute founder and sinker cases.

This measurement helps you monitor the horse's progress and **along with type of founder** (Laminitis, Acute, Chronic Type I, Sinker and Chronic Type II), aids in helping estimate the prognosis and probability of return to soundness. Further discussion of this measurement will be covered in Chapter 4.

Angle S (figure 3.2)

Angle S is the angle between the dorsal hoof wall and the ground.

Angle T (figure 3.2)

Angle T is the angle between the dorsal cortex of the distal phalanx and the ground.

Angle U (figure 3.2)

Angle U is the angle between a line connecting the centers of curvature of the proximal distal interphanlangeal joints and the ground.

Angle of Hoof Capsule Rotation (figure 3.2)

This is Angle T minus Angle S.

Hoof capsule rotation is a poor prognostic indicator of the outcome and success of treatment. Further discussion of this topic will be covered in Chapter 4.

Angle of Distal Phalanx Rotation (figure 3.2)

This is Angle T minus Angle U.

The angle of distal phalanx rotation helps you determine how much foot should be trimmed to realign the hoof capsule and phalangeal axis.

A **positive number** or increased angle indicates the amount of heel to be removed in order to align the phalangeal axis. A **negative number** or decreased angle indicates the amount of heel to be raised in order to align the phalangeal axis.

It is wise to do a toe-wedge test first in horses with excessive heel to remove, due to the possibility of contracted tendons.

Some horses will grow an excessive amount of heel due to shortening of the distance between the origin and insertion of the deep digital flexor muscle-tendon unit. What this means for the farrier is one cannot entirely correct the phalanx angle by lowering the heels, as they would do normally.

Excessive lowering of the heels in a horse that tests positive with a toe-wedge test, will make the horse very lame as the muscle-tendon unit is stretched.

In order to perform a toe-wedge test, simply place about 10 degrees of wedge pads under the toe of the foot. Lift the opposite limb so the horse stands on the leg with the toe wedges, for a period of 30 to 60 seconds.

You may have a case of contracture if the horse becomes more uncomfortable or the tendon becomes very tight, when compared to the non-wedged foot. Do not remove the heel.

The farrier will have to leave more heel than they would like until assessed by the veterinarian. In these cases, the author has had success after the veterinarian prescribed **Methocarbamol (Robaxin ™),** a skeletal muscle relaxant.

In such contracture cases, the author removed as much heel as possible and reset the shoes every week, removing a little more heel each time, until the phalanx angle is correct.

If the horse does not respond to the muscle relaxant, another alternative may be for the veterinarian to transect the inferior check ligament or the deep digital flexor tendon.

Frog Plate Placement Calculation (F) (figure 3.2)

This is the distance between the tack (which is merely a reference point to determine the proper placement of the frog plate), and a line drawn perpendicular to the ground, immediately behind the extensor process and bisecting the coffin joint space.

In my opinion, **this is the easiest and most accurate** way to calculate this measurement. It is essential that you **use radiographs and not guessing**, to establish the frog plate placement. A frog plate placed too far forward can increase pain, decrease blood flow through the paracuneal artery and allow the distal phalanx to have a more levering effect. One placed too far back will not provide proper biomechanical support.

A second method for determining frog plate placement is to measure the length of the solar margin of the distal phalanx and them measure back 37% from the tip of the distal phalanx. This method doesn't work well when the distal phalanx is degenerating.

I would suggest being familiar with both methods as a means of checks and balances.

Shoe Toe Placement Calculation (ST) (figure 3.2)

This is the distance between the tack (which is merely a reference point to determining the proper placement of the toe of the shoe), and a line drawn parallel to the dorsal aspect of the distal phalanx, at the normal wall thickness measurement (L x 0.25 or uncorrected for magnification at 13-15 mm for ponies, 15-17 mm for horses and 17-19 mm for draft breeds).

In my opinion, this is the easiest and most accurate way to determine the proper placement of the toe of the heart bar shoe.

The farrier will then remove the distorted hoof, exposing the laminar wedge. The author finds this method easier, more accurate, supportive and cost effective than removing the dorsal hoof wall first, before applying the heart bar shoe.

A shoe placed too far forward will not allow the farrier to remove enough distorted toe. A shoe placed to far back will cause the farrier to dangerously remove too much toe.

Other Concurrent Problems

At the bottom of each form is a place to document other concurrent problems that may or may not be related to the foundering incident. This may include observations such as: Abscesses, Serum Pockets, Infectious Osteitis, Pedal Osteitis, Osteomyelitis, Keratomas, dropped Soles, Prolapsed Soles, Ringbone, Sidebones, Fractures, etc...

Chapter 4

How to Determine Prognosis

and the chances
the horse will return to soundness

Hoof Capsule Rotation

Although used by many veterinarians and farriers, **hoof capsule rotation is a poor prognostic indicator** of the outcome and success of treatment. The author has had horse's with 35 degrees of rotation survive and return to soundness, while other horses with 5 degrees of rotation may never attain better than pasture soundness.

Figure 4.1 illustrates how meaningless hoof capsule rotation is in terms of describing and making prognostic judgements.

In these examples, the hoof capsule rotation are both 10 degrees. Assuming these are acute or Chronic Type I cases, the one on the left may only need a foot dressing while the one on the right may need a more extreme treatment.

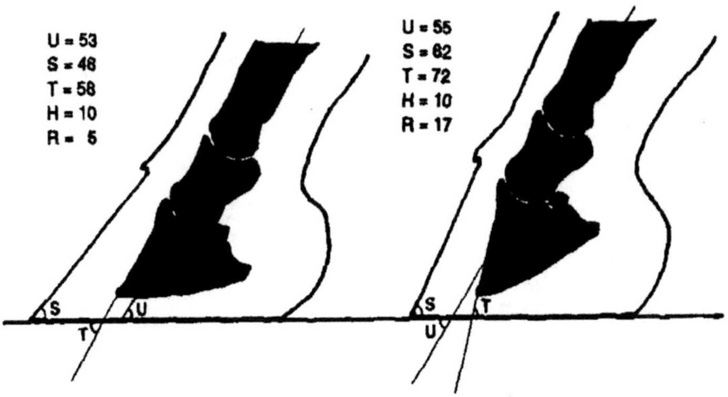

Figure 4.1 - Illustration by Robert Eustace, BVSc, Cert EO, Cert EP. FRCVS, showing how meaningless hoof capsule rotation is in describing and prognosticating founder case (used by permission).

One of my favorite quotes concerning rotation comes from Colorado's **George Platt, DVM**, who specializes in foundered horses. He states, *" I don't care about the degree of rotation. Its like pregnancy, either you are or you aren't. If they are rotated they're probably foundered."*

Robert Eustace, BVSc, Cert EO, Cert EP, FRCVS, who also specializes in foundered horse states, *"hoof capsule rotation is insignificant and meaningless in terms of describing and making prognostic statements."*

Pain Level, Breed, Gender, Age

The author and other's research findings have shown that the horse's age, gender, breed, number of feet affected or pain level, showed any correlation to the chances of survival or return to soundness.

Founder Distance

A method for Acute and Sinker founders is to use the founder distance method and chart developed by **Robert Eustace, BVSc, Cert EO, Cert EP, FWCVS.** The chart can help aid in the predication of recovery (figure 4.2).

Robert Eustace, BVSc, Cert EO, Cert EP, FWCVS, writes, *"Although the conclusions which can be drawn from the graph should not be regarded as being cast in tablets of stone, the measurement of founder distance represents a more scientific basis on which to make decisions on the life or death of foundered horses."*

The author has found that the greater the founder distance for any type of founder, the less chance the horse will return to soundness. The author has had horses with founder distances as great as 18.5 mm return to their previous soundness. However, the chances of returning to soundness are greater if the founder distance is less.

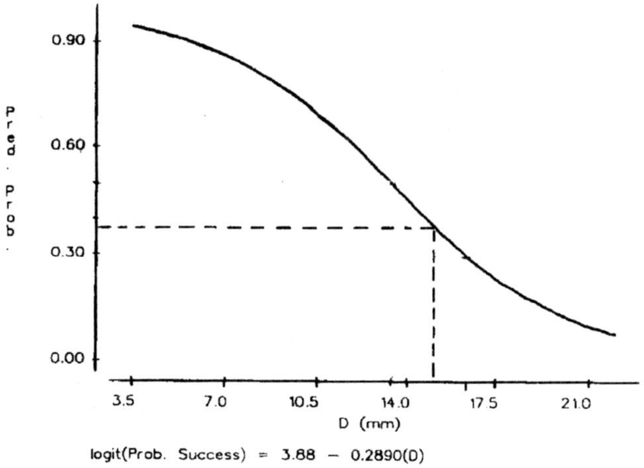

Figure 4.2 - Founder Distance Chart from data collected by Robert A. Eustace, BVSc, Cert EO, Cert EP, FWCVS, (used by permission).

As supported by the author's research, the best use of the founder distance is to compare measurements from the original radiograph. The faster the founder distance returns to normal, the more likely the horse will return to previous soundness, as there will be less damage to the foot. For instance, and Acute foundered horse originally has a 9 mm founder distance and four weeks late at the resetting, the horse has a 4.5 mm founder distance. This horse is exhibiting a rapid recovery from the founder.

Founder Types

Based on the works of **Robert Eustace, BVSc, Cert EO, Cert EP, FWCVS, the author and others;** identifying the type of founder the horse is experiencing is a very good, if not the best, predicator of determining the chances that the horse will return to soundness.

It is important that these **different types** of founder can be recognized, **as each carries a different prognosis** and each can be expected to respond to treatments differently. The five types are Laminitis, Acute, Chronic Type I, Sinker and Chronic Type II.

In chapter 5, the author will discuss when you have two different types of founder in the same horse. In some cases, due to weight bearing, a more severe founder develops in the originally unaffected weight bearing foot. However, the author has found that most have **limb length disparities** and shoes them accordingly.

First, let us consider and discuss what a normal radiographic foot should look like (figure 4.3).

In the normal foot, the phalanges are in a straight line. The dorsal hoof wall hoof wire marker is parallel to the front of the distal phalanx. The top of the wire is in a normal position just above the extensor process of the distal phalanx. The solar surface of the distal phalanx is at a normal 5-10 degree angle to the ground surface.

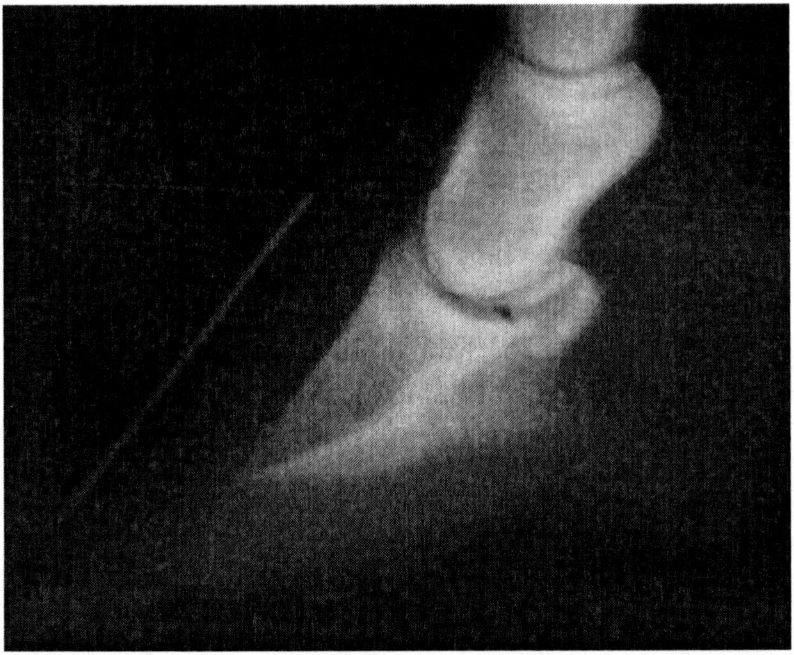

Figure 4.3 - Lateromedial radiographic view of a normal foot.

In the Acute foundered horse (figure 4.4), the distal phalanx has started to move down and backward within the foot.

It is critical to understand that before a hoof rotates, the wall thickness increases; then the distal phalanx descends. Being able to identify this by the radiographs and getting treatment started early can make all the difference in the recovery of the horse.

There is an increased vertical distance between the top of the dorsal hoof wall wire marker and the top of the extensor process of the distal phalanx (founder distance). Next, there is loss of parallelism between the dorsal hoof wall wire marker and the dorsal aspect of the distal phalanx.

Palpation of the dorsal coronary band can reveal a slight depression in the skin just above the hoof wall. The depression indicates that the laminae within the foot has separated and the distal phalanx is moving distally within the hoof capsule.

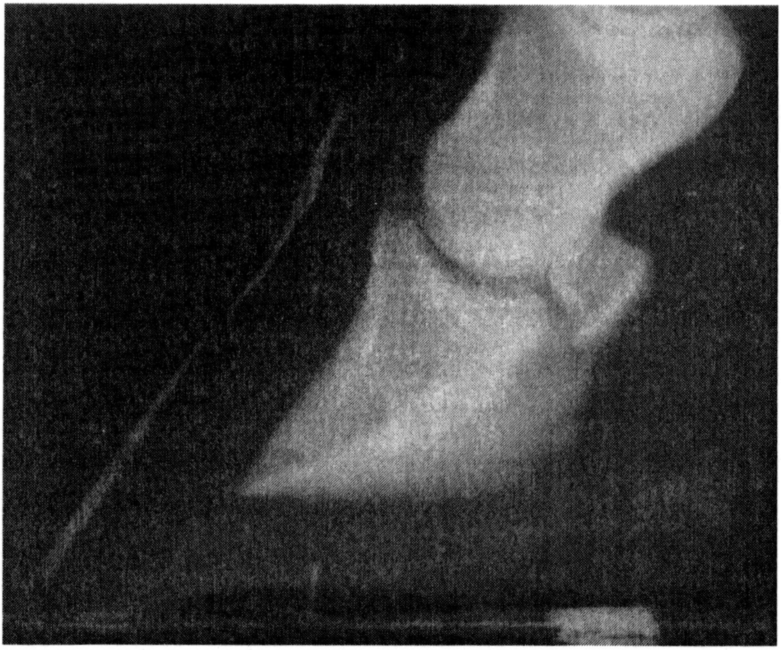

Figure 4.4 - Lateromedial radiographic view of an Acute foundered foot.

In the **Chronic Type I** foundered horse (figure 4.5), the phalangeal axis is not straight, but can be easily corrected by lowering the heels. The toe is overgrown, and new horn at the top of the foot is nearly parallel with the dorsal aspect of the distal phalanx. Also, the toe of the hoof may be dished.

In the **Sinker** (figure 4.6), the founder distance is greatly increased compared to normal. The tip of the distal phalanx is resting on the inside of the sole causing it to become convex. The sole may be prolapsed (dropped sole) or the distal phalanx may have penetrated out through the sole. Palpation of the coronet reveals a distinct depression, which extends from one heel around to the other heel.

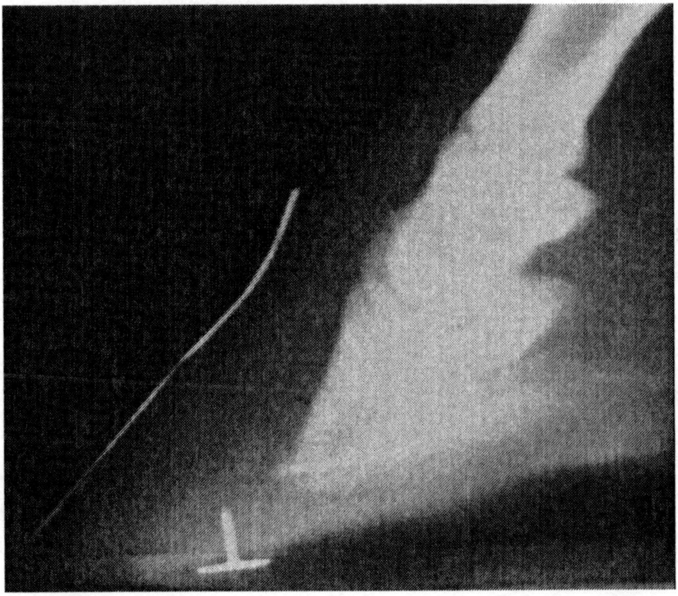

Figure 4.5 - Lateromedial radiographic view of a Chronic Type I foundered foot.

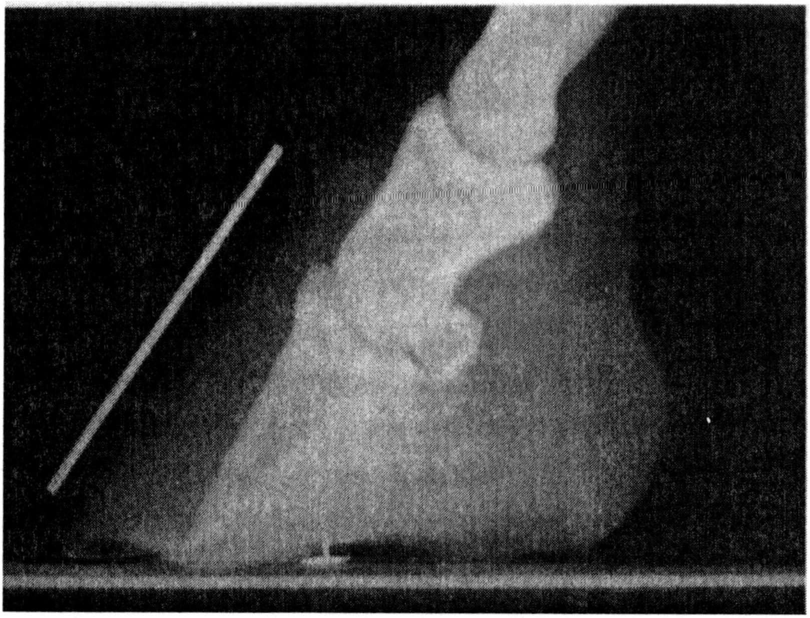

Figure 4.6 - Lateromedial radiographic view of a Sinker foot.

In the **Chronic Type II** foundered horse (figure 4.7), part of the distal phalanx has remodeled. There may be active **Infectious Osteitis** (commonly, but mistakenly called Osteomyelitis) that could require surgery but rarely helps and has a very poor prognosis. In these cases, the overgrown toe is a solid wedge of laminar horn right up to the coronary band.

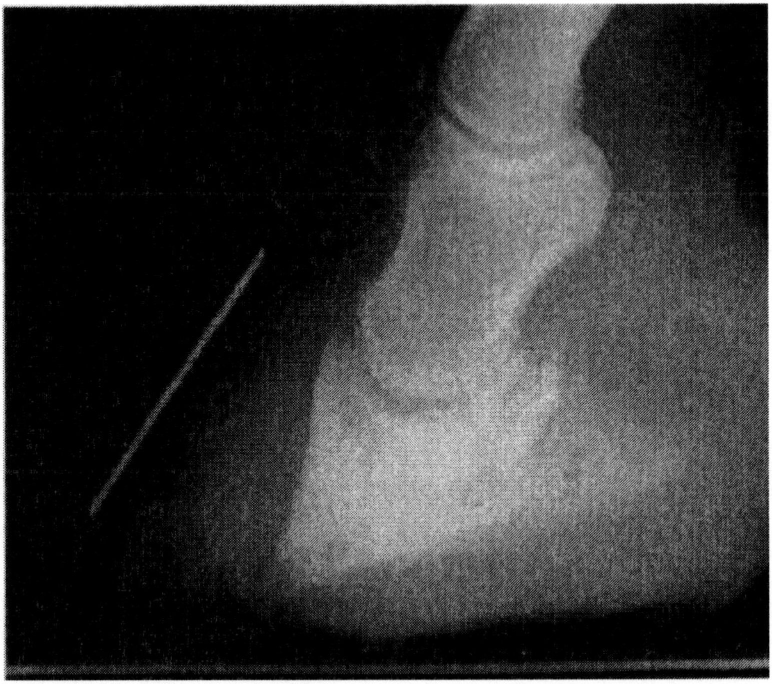

Figure 4.7 - Lateromedial radiographic view of a Chronic Type II foundered foot.

Based on the type of founder, the expected success rates from the works of **Robert Eustace, BVSc, Cert EO, Cert EP, FRCVS**, are shown below.

Expected Success Rates Based on Founder Type (1998)

by
Robert A. Eustace, BVSc, Cert EO, Cert EP, FRCVS

77% returned to original soundness

23% were destroyed or were unable to be ridden

Laminitis - 100%

Acute Founder - 82%

Chronic Founder - 78%

Sinker - 20%

Based on the type of founder, the expected success rates from the works of **the author**, are shown below.

Expected Survival and Return to Useful Soundness Rates Based on Type of Founder (2003)

© 2003 by Esco Buff, PhD, CF

Over a 12 year period from 1991 to 2003,
627 new-foundered cases were treated

98% survived (616)
82% returned to original soundness (514)
18 % did not return to original soundness (113)
Of these, 16% were pasture sound (102)
and 2% were euthanized (11)

Laminitis
100% survival rate
100% returned to original soundness

Acute
100% survival rate
100% returned to original soundness

Chronic Type I
100% survival rate
96% returned to original soundness

Sinker
99% survival rate
69% returned to original soundness

Chronic Type II
99% survival rate
53% returned to original soundness

Remember, the reasons for **higher success rates are due** to the veterinarian and farrier successfully working together, and by the application of correct rigid (non-adjustable) heart bar shoes.

Founder is a systemic disease resulting from a stress triggering insult. It is the **role of the veterinarian** to diagnosis the insult, if at all possible, and provide treatment for the insult and any other systemic problems. It is the **role of the farrier** to provide immediate and correct biomechanical support of the bone column.

We now have a completed **Founder Data Collection and Analysis Form** © (figure 4.8). We also know the type of founder and the founder distance.

From the data collected, we now have significant information to provide the horse owner, to establish a prognosis and to perform treatment. From the data, the horse owner will either have the team provide treatment or not. In most cases, the horse owner must make substantial commitments of both time and money.

Treatment will take months to restore the damaged hoof. Each case will be different and will require good nursing and aftercare.

FOUNDER DATA COLLECTION AND ANALYSIS FORM

Owner Alice Reed

Veterinarian LEVC

Farrier Esco Buff

Horse Emmy

Breed Paint/Pinto

Gender Mare Age 1988

Date of Radiograph 8/21/03

Date of Data Collection 8/22/03

(Front) Hind

(Left) Right

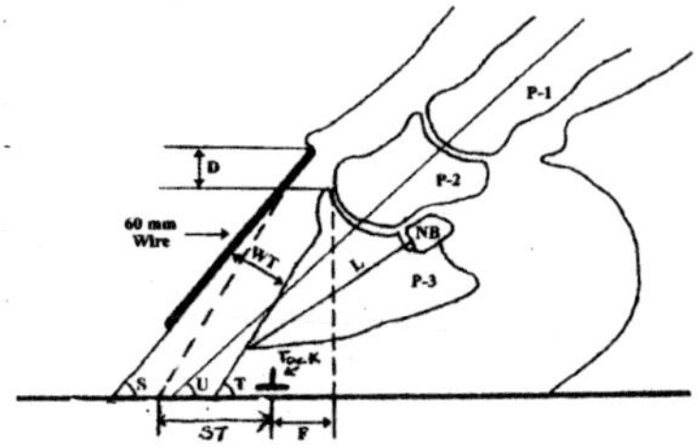

Wire Length

Actual = 76 mm

Radiologically = 83 mm

Founder Type

Laminitis (Acute) CT-I CT-II Sinker

Magnification Correction = Length Measured Radiographically X Actual Wire Length / Radiographic Wire Length

= 0.9156 mm

= 0.92 mm

Angle S (Dorsal Wall Angle) = 57 degrees

Angle T (P-3 Angle) = 67 degrees

Angle U (Phalanx Angle) = 67 degrees

Angle of Hoof Capsule Rotation = Angle T (67) minus Angle S (57) = 10 degrees

Angle of Distal Phalanx Rotation = Angle T (67) minus Angle U (67) = 0 degrees

L (Palmer Cortex of the Distal Phalanx Distance)

Radiologically = 58 mm

Corrected for Magnification = 53.4 mm

F (Frog Plate Placement Calculation)

Radiologically = 35 mm

Corrected for Magnification = 32.2 mm

WT (Wall Thickness)

Radiologically = 25 mm

Corrected for Magnification = 23 mm

Normal Wall Thickness (L x .25) = 13.3 mm

ST (Shoe Toe Placement Calculation)

Radiologically = 78 mm

Corrected for Magnification = 71.8 mm

D (Founder Distance)

Radiologically = 11 mm

Corrected for Magnification = 10.1 mm

Veterinarian/Farrier Treatment to Date and Any Other Concurrent Problems:
(Abscess, Serum Pockets, Infectious Osteitis, Pedal Osteitis, Osteomyelitis, Dropped Sole, Prolapsed Sole, Ringbone, Sidebones....)

Dorsal hoof wall crack

Figure 4.8 - A completed Founder Data Collection and Analysis Form©.

Chapter
5

Shoeing the Foundered Horse

how to use the radiograph to successfully shoe the foundered horse

The goal of shoeing is to counteract the downward movement of the distal phalanx. This can be done most effectively through the use of heart bar shoes.

Heart bar shoes should be applied as soon as possible to help stabilize the bone column. The stabilizing effect of support via of controlled pressure on the frog, helps arrest the founder damage.

The author finds that nailing a rigid heart bar shoe onto horses in any stage of laminitis and founder will provide immediate relief. However, some animals may be in too much pain or not enough foot remains to apply a shoe with nails. In such cases, glue-on heart bar shoes provide an alternative for the farrier.

Do not fit heart bar shoes to horses that have received an analgesic. Such horses will be less sensitive and the farrier will not be able to assess the response to excessive frog pressure.

First, transfer the data from the form to the foot.

On the foot, the position of the tack has already been marked during the radiograph process (figure 5.1)

Now mark the magnification corrected frog plate or "F" calculation on the frog (figure 5.1).

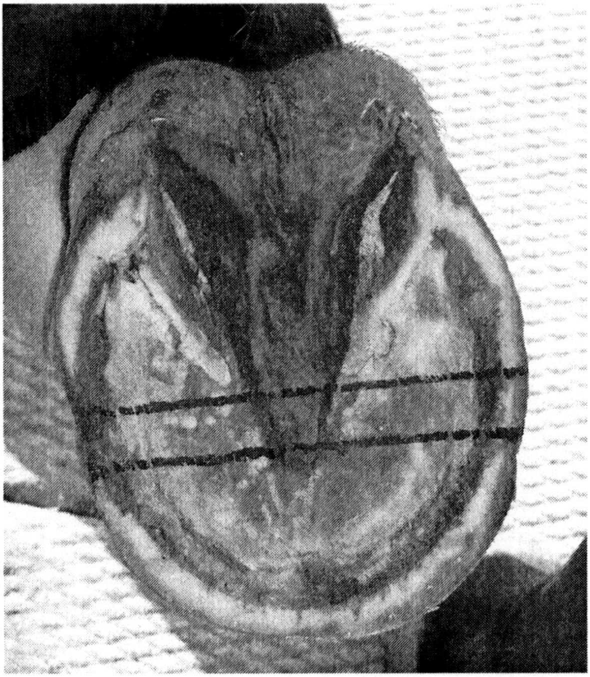

Figure 5.1 - Solar view of tack marker line and "F" marker line

From here, there are a couple of ways to figure out where the **toe of your heart bar shoe** should end. The author would suggest you use the normal hoof wall thickness method until you get more experienced shoeing foundered horses.

For this method, draw a parallel line on the radiograph to the dorsal aspect of the distal phalanx, at a distance of 13-15 mm for a pony, 15-17 mm for a horse or 17-19 mm for a draft (uncorrected for magnification (figure 5.2). Measure from the tack to where this line intersects the sole and correct for magnification.

Now take this measurement or "ST" calculation to the horse and mark this location on the bottom of the foot. This is the spot where the toe of the shoe will end (figure 5.3).

The exception to this rule is with Laminitic or Acute foundered horses. For these cases, shoe to the toe of the hoof. Remember, a horse that is foundering first shows signs of increasing hoof wall thickness, then dropping distance, before rotation occurs.

In many Acute foundered cases, the author has seen return to normal hoof wall thickness and dropping distance measurements within four week. **You don't want to be over zealous with the rasp in these cases.**

We now have the reference points marked on the foot and are ready to make the heart bar shoe.

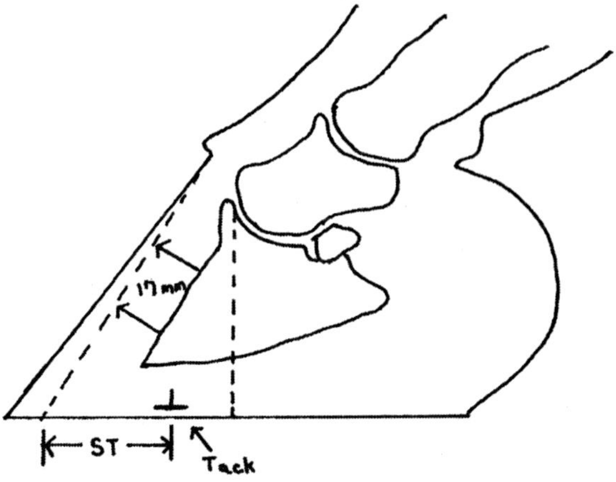

Figure 5.2 - Drawing showing the shoe toe placement calculation (ST).

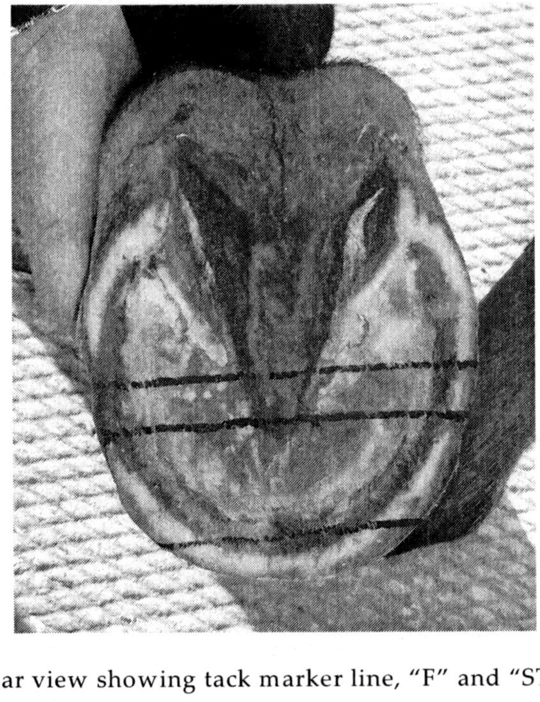

Figure 5.3 - Solar view showing tack marker line, "F" and "ST" spots.

There are many ways to make a heart bar shoe. The most accurate, efficient and cost-effective method is best used. For these reason, the author prefers to fit a standard rim shoe and forge the frog plate out of round stock (figure 5.4).

The frog plate is then welded into the heels of the rim shoe at the same plane as the frog (figure 5.5).

If not enough pressure against the frog is obtained, the farrier can rivet a frog pad of correct thickness to the frog plate. An alternative method is to drill several holes in your frog plate and apply a layer of adhesive, such as **Adhere ™ or Superfast ™ (Vettec, Inc).** After the adhesive has dried, rasp it down to the desired thickness (figure 5.6 and 5.7). The author has used both methods successfully without complications.

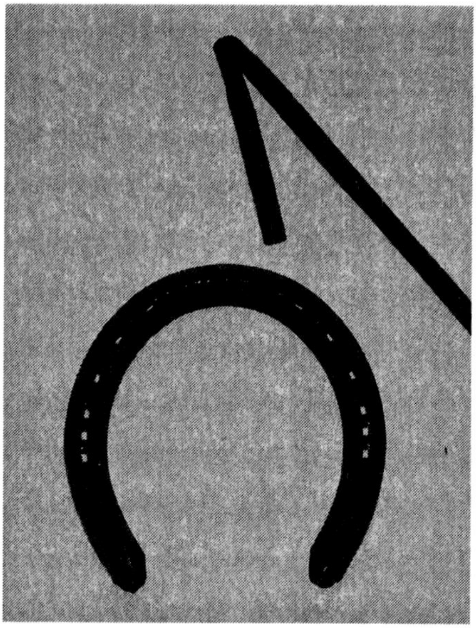

Figure 5.4 - A rim shoe and forged heart bar insert.

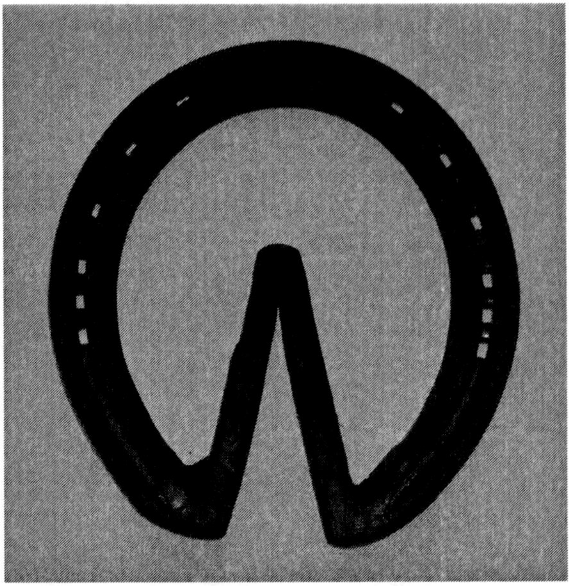

Figure 5.5 - A finished correct heart bar shoe.

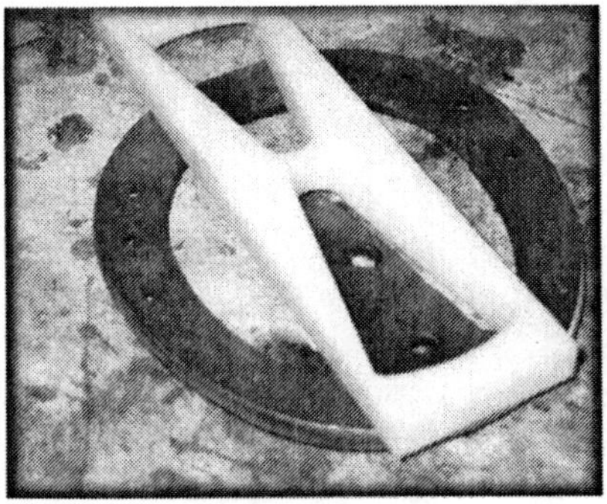

Figure 5.6 - Heart bar shoe ready for Superfast ™ with the aid of the Heartbar Mold from Vettec, Inc.

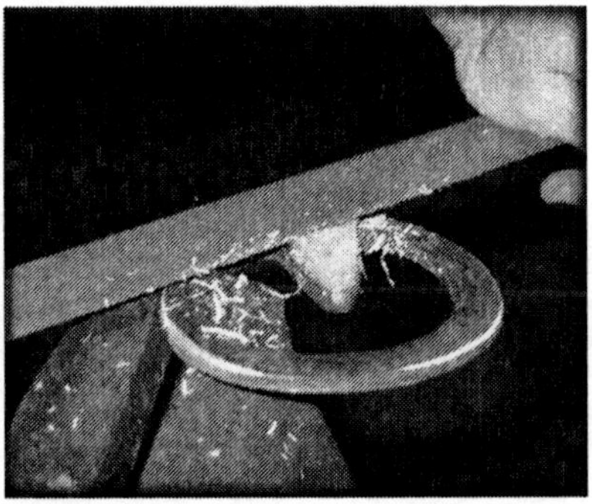

Figure 5.7 - Rasping down the adhesive to the desired thickness.

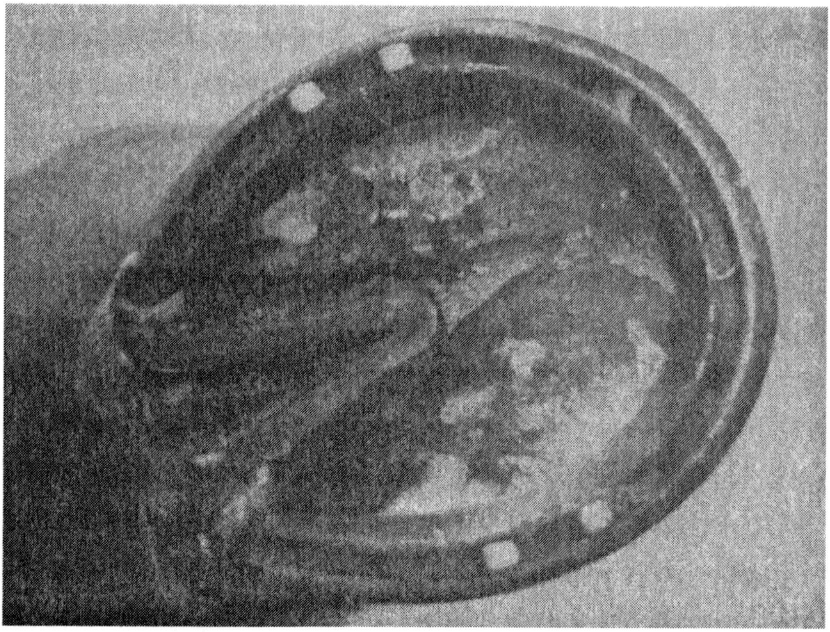

Figure 5.8 - Solar view of a correctly placed and shod heart bar shoe on a foundered foot.

Heart bar shoes should be slightly longer than the hoof in order to give adequate support to the bone column. Also, the toe of the shoe should be the same shape as the coffin bone's shape.

There should be **no sole pressure**. Rim pads may be needed to increase the distance from the sole to the shoe. **Hospital plates are often necessary and may be useful to prevent environmental sole pressure.** Nails should be located behind the point of the frog plate in order to avoid further damage to the laminae.

The frog **must be visible** on all sides and in front of the frog plate to prevent constriction of the paracuneal artery (figure 5.8 and 5.9).

A guideline is to ensure at least 1/8" of frog visible around the frog plate. The tip of the frog plate is placed at the "F" calculation measurement.

If you marked the hoof correctly, the only real variable in shoeing with heart bars becomes the amount of frog pressure.

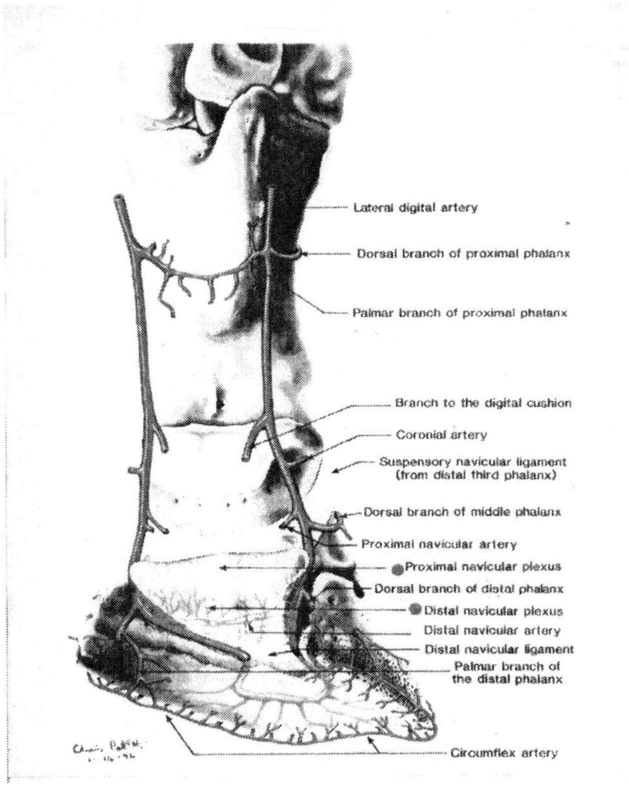

Figure 5.9 - Blood flow chart by Christopher C. Pollitt, BVSc, PhD, (used by permission).

It is wise to use a hoof tester to evaluate the sensitivity of the frog. Occasionally, the frog is too sensitive to put pressure up to the "F" point and you will have to shorten your heart bar frog plate. Sore frogs may be due to previous excessive frog support or due to fluid accumulation beneath the frog and sole.

The pressure placed against the frog by the heart bar is determined by feel. The shoe should be squeezed down against the frog by the thumbs. The force required to resist the frog and rest the shoe on the wall is about right for most horses. Usually this distance is about 1/8".

The frog plate should be made so when the shoe is nailed on, there is equal pressure on the hoof wall and frog, in order to prevent pressure necrosis.

Tack on the shoe with two nails and allow the horse to bear weight, watching for signs of discomfort. Resting the opposite foot or a big sigh of relief as the horse loads the shod foot are good signs. Starting to load the foot then backing off and resting it, as well as developing tension around the mouth, are bad signs.

The shoe must be removed and the frog plate readjusted until it provides the correct support, before you finish nailing the shoe onto the hoof.

The distorted hoof should be rasped down to the same shape as the toe of the shoe, exposing the laminar wedge. Remember, the exception is for horse suffering from Laminitis and Acute founder (figure 5.10).

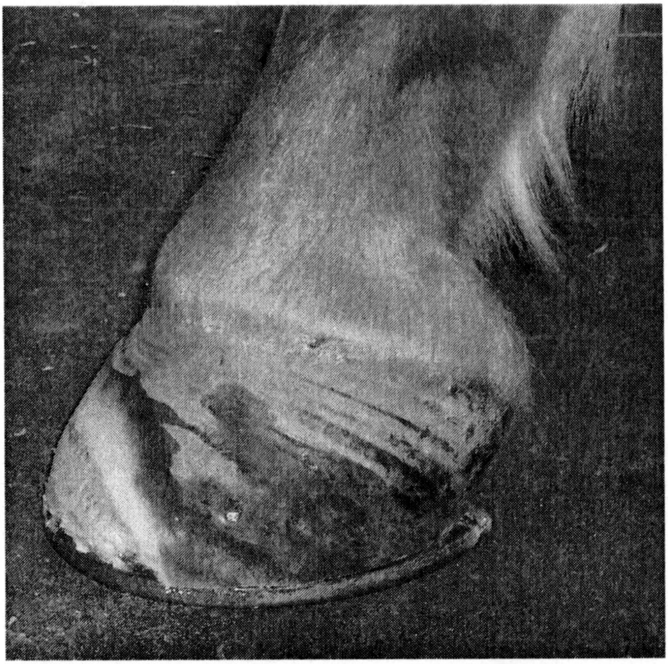

Figure 5.10 - Weight bearing on the newly applied steel heart bar shoe.

Further resection may be needed in the advent of abscess formation.

Abscesses in foundered horses should not be drained by opening the sole, but rather through the dorsal hoof wall. This will keep the sole stronger as well as prevent the swollen solar corium from prolapsing through the opening.

The author treats any abscesses with sugardine (a paste created by mixing Betadine ® and sugar). Ichthammol 20% or magna paste can be use on the coronary band to draw out exudates (figure 5.11).

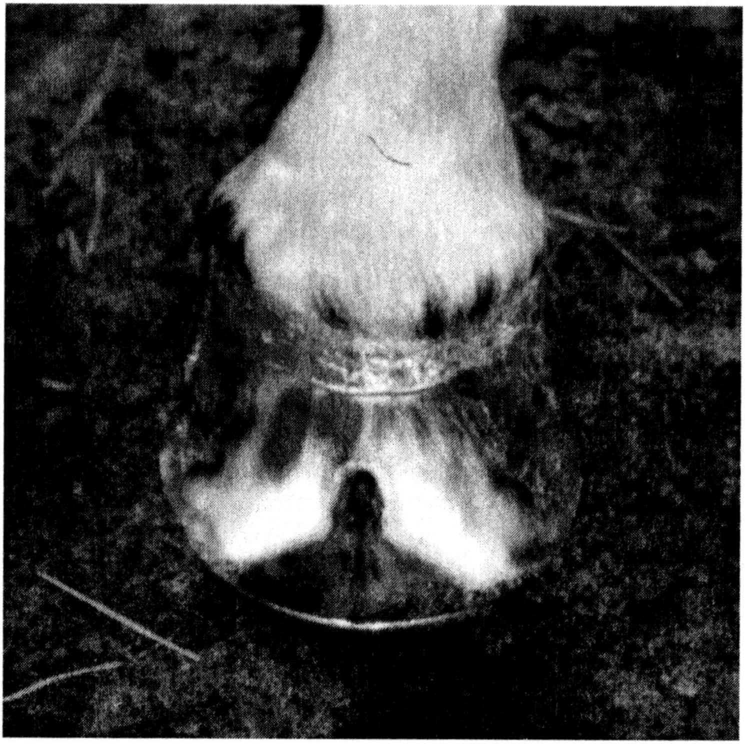

Figure 5.11 - Abscess on a foundered horse being drained through the dorsal hoof wall.

The author occasionally performs hoof wall resections. These are usually warranted when you need to remove detached dorsal hoof wall, allow drainage of abscesses, debride any necrotic laminae, and to relieve the upward pressure on the coronary plexus by the hoof wall migration (figure 5.12).

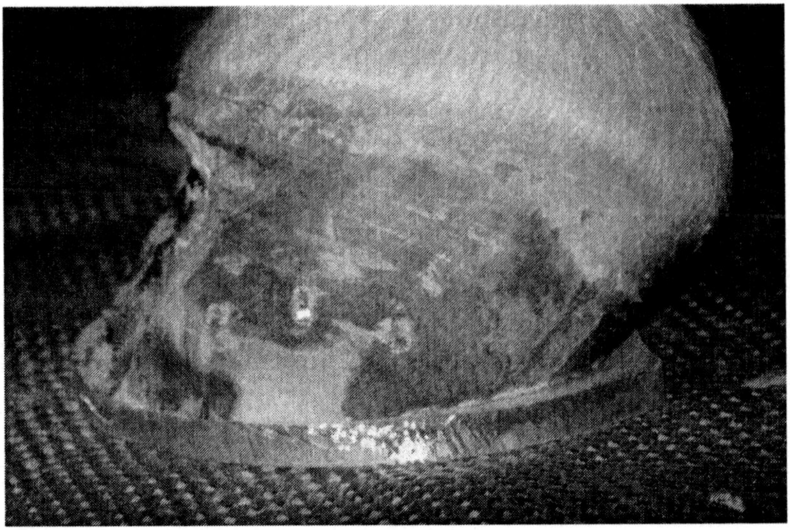

Figure 5.12 - Hoof wall resection on a foundered horse.

Resections are usually a bloodless procedure performed by the farrier and/or the veterinarian. The procedure doesn't usually require sedation, but does require veterinary supervision. In these cases, the farrier may also have to add side or T-clips to the shoe in order to help better stabilize the hoof capsule.

Remember, a properly fitted heart bar shoe transfers part of the weight bearing capacity of the foot to the frog, thus allowing other parts of the foot to be rehabilitated.

The author recommends heart bar shoes to be reset at intervals not to exceed four weeks. In the early stages of treatment, the heels will outgrow the toe and it will be essential to trim and shoe for correct heart bar placement. The heart bar shoes should be applied until the feet have stabilized, grown new hoof wall, and the horse is comfortable while walking.

As the horse progressively becomes better, you apply less and less frog pressure until no frog pressure has been applied for a period of one or two shoeings. When the horse is sound and healing is progressing well, the author usually puts the horse into an aluminum bar shoe. As the new hoof wall growth reaches the ground level, the author applies regular shoes.

Shoeing the Foundered Limb Length Disparity horse

Limb length disparity is an observable body imbalance and physical deviation that has been created due to injuries, congenital, hereditary, environmental, muscular and/or spinal problems.

Identifying limb length disparities should be done by a qualified farrier and veterinarian and will include a thorough evaluation of the conformation, muscles, skeletal structures, movement, and attitude of the horse.

Shoeing limb length disparities can be challenging.

The front shorter leg has a hoof that is more narrow than the opposite hoof and is sometimes called a club foot. The hoof will also have more heel than the opposite hoof.

The front longer leg has a hoof that is wider than the opposite hoof and is sometimes called a platter foot. The hoof will also be more underrun than the opposite hoof.

The pectoral muscles and dorsal scapular ligaments at the shoulder will not be symmetrical. The alignment of the medial distal radial malleoses in the front legs and the chestnuts in the hind legs will not be even.

The horse could be suffering from a subluxation of the sacro-iliac joint and **a qualified chiropractic veterinarian should be considered.**

The goal of shoeing a foundered limb length disparity horse is to cause the horse to be more comfortable, reduce pain and stress, and equalize weight bearing. To accomplish this, **the farrier and veterinarian must understand** that problems in the upper body can create symptoms in the legs and feet.

The foundered limb length disparity horse usually exhibits two different founder types. Generally the shorter front leg will almost always have a more severe founder than the longer front leg. An example could be that the longer leg will be suffering from acute founder while the shorter leg from a sinker. Or, the longer leg will be a Chronic Type I and the shorter leg a Chronic Type II.

Also, the solar surface of the distal phalanx on the longer front limb will usually be far less than the normal 5-10 degree angle to the ground surface.

Apply a lift rim pad on the front foot of the shorter leg. If the longer leg has a broken back pastern axis, apply a rim wedge pad to correct the angle.

Shoeing the hind legs of a limb length disparity horse requires a higher level of farrier assessment skill and should be avoided if the farrier lacks this knowledge. However, the farrier would generally apply a rim wedge pad on the hind leg that travels under the body. In the absence of a chiropractic veterinarian, this will alleviate much of the muscular pain associated with the subluxation of the sacro-iliac joint, but will not correct the problem.

The late **Tony Gonzales** has written, *"Admittedly, lifting a horse will look bizarre. People don't like bizarre and they don't like standing around listening to the rationale behind the methods that seem strange."*

Remember, the goal of shoeing the foundered limb length disparity horse is to put the horse back in balance in order to cause the horse to be more comfortable. The horse is already going through a challenging, stressful, painful time with being foundered; and doesn't need this compounded by their limb length disparity.

Chapter 6

Final Words

and aftercare instructions

Proper **aftercare is critical** and includes resetting the shoes on a frequent basis by an experienced, qualified farrier, regular examinations by the veterinarian and re-bandaging and exercising by the horse owner.

It has been the authors experience, as well as many others, that the **heart bar shoe has the greatest chance of success** compared with other options for the treatment of foundered horses.

Many people who say heart bar shoes don't work haven't taken the time to learn how to apply them correctly.

The late **Burney Chapman, CJF** who introduced the heart bar shoe at the 1983 American Farriers Association Convention and the 1984 American Association of Equine Practitioners Convention said, *"There are more wrong ways than right ways to use it."*

The heart bar shoe must be constructed, fit and applied with accuracy.

Bernard Pelletier has said, *"Heart bar shoes are a canvas for creativity and when they are used correctly, they are the keys to soundness for thousands of horses that would otherwise be retired, or worse. There are still widespread errors in the fitting and application of these shoes, and almost 30 years after Burney Chapman brought them to our attention; they are still the dangerous, double-edged sword of the farrier world. Once mastered, they can be the professional's Excalibur.*
With a little knowledge and training, a farrier can save many foundered horse with these "Excalibur Shoes."

Most horse are immediately more comfortable with correctly fitted heart bar shoes.

The late **Burney Chapman, CJF** wrote, *"due to the complex anatomy of the vascular system of the equine foot, care must be given as to what king of treatment and devices are use to stabilize the foundering foot."*

The author and others have also found many devices for shoeing foundered horses that do not work, work with little consistency or cause more pain for the horse than doing nothing at all.

Some of these devices are (Chapman, Platt, 1984):

- The egg bar/straight bar shoe, which has no stabilizing effect on the bone column.

- The reverse shoe, which gives no stabilization to the distal phalanx and leave s the toe exposed.

- A shoe that raises the heel and takes stress off the deep digital flexor tendon, which aligns all the laminae parallel to the ground, causing the bone column to sink. Raising the heels can also be detrimental to the distal aspect of the distal phalanx.

- Styrofoam ™ pads, which give no stability to the bone column and once the heels settle into the foam, provide sole pressure, thus destroying the blood supply.

- Any pad on the foot surface of the shoe, except rim, with or without packing, as it gives no stability to the bone column and can provide sole pressure, thus destroying the blood supply. The exception would be with a horse with big frogs and full arches.

Exercise

During recovery, the horse owner **should not force exercise** the horse. At one time, exercise was thought to be beneficial by increasing blood flow to the foot. There is already a tremendous increase in blood flow to the foot, however **there is nominal perfusion** of the dermal laminae. Exercise will not improve this situation, but rather will mechanically tear the remaining laminae making the founder worse.

Continue to stall the horse in a box stall with at least ten to twelve inches of bedding. Restrict the horse to stall rest until the horse has recovered enough to walk around without analgesics and without lameness.

Next, I would suggest **leisure hand walking**, twice daily, for fifteen to twenty minutes at a time. From this point on, exercise should be determined based on how well the horse is progressing with recovery.

Effects of the Triggering Event

There are a number of reasons or causes for laminitis and founder. Understanding what was the triggering event will be helpful in the aftercare treatment of the horse.

One time triggering events such as grass colic, grain overloads, road founder... can be dealt with effectively. Recovery proceeds faster once the horse has been removed from the triggering event.

Metabolic problems such as Cushings Disease, abnormal thyroid functions, equine metabolic syndrome and severe infectious or inflammatory diseases will require additional recovery time. Once on proper medication and diet, the body requires time to stabilize, and the triggering event is still playing a part in the foundered horse.

Medications

The author, along with other farriers and veterinarians, have discovered many medication regimes are counter productive, useless or harmful in treating founder.

Systemic Antibiotics may be prescribed. However, they may not be effective for the treatment of hoof infections because of decreased blood flow to the affected tissues.

Anti-inflammatories, such as **phenylbutazone (bute)**, are contraindicated. These drugs mask the symptoms of the founder pain causing additional damage to the laminae by not allowing the horse to rest or shift their weight between limbs.

Some people are more interested in providing pain relief than saving the animal. Pain helps prevent further damage to the affected area. Rest it! Another favorite quote of the authors originates from **George Platt, DVM**. *"My pain relief is the heart bar shoe."* The author has found this statement to be profound and true.

Vasodilator drugs, such as **Isoxuprine**, are used to relax the blood vessels. Although this drug is unlikely to be harmful, it has failed to increase capsular blood flow and is contraindicated in Chronic Type II founder cases as it increase the rate of resorption of the distal phalanx.

As of today, I know of **no specific medication** that will return the blood flow to normal.

Feeding

The author recommends feeding the horse a good quality grass hay and hoof supplement such as **Farrier's Formula®.**

The author can't emphasize enough the importance of feeding a high quality supplement, especially when coupled with correct shoeing principles.

Let's take a moment to discuss available feed supplements. Many products report improvement in hoof quality. The author has researched and tried many of these products with little or no success.

The author has experienced excellent results with one specific feed supplement that stimulates rapid hoof growth. This feed supplement is **Life Data Labs ®,**
Farrier's Formula ®.

Farrier's Formula ® is a hoof supplement based on conclusive scientific research published in referred journals. Rival manufacturer's unsupported claims for products directly imitating **Farrier's Formula ®** should be questioned.

Life Data Labs, Inc. ® is and ISO 9001 certified company affirming that the company's manufacturing operation adheres to a internationally recognized quality of standards.

The commitment required to earn and maintain ISO 9001 certification shows Life Data Lab's, Inc. ® desire to consistently provide quality products. The ISO system required that Life Dat Labs, Inc. ® maintain **laboratory proof of potency,** and thereby freshness. Likewise, Farrier's Formula ® is correctly packaged and dated for freshness.

Farrier's Formula ® is the only product that has been independently researched and tested. Also, it remains the number one recommended hoof supplement by United States farriers for eleven consecutive years.

Many horses experience metabolic disease stress and during founder episodes, will require a proven, quality supplement. **Farrier's Formula** ® contains the correct balance of important supplements such as L-tyrosine, iodine and Phenylalanine for such horses.

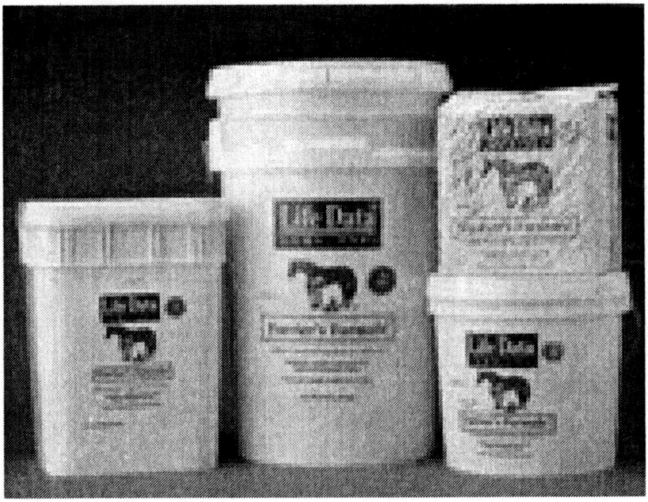

Figure 6.1 - Life Data Labs, Inc. ® Products (used by permission).

Resource Guide and References

American Farriers Association 27th Annual Convention Official Program,
Lessiter Publications, Inc, Brookfield, Wisconsin,
page 75-8, 1998.

Animal Nutrition Products,
by Life Data Labs, Inc. ®,
Cherokee, Alabama, 2003.

Blood Flow Chart (figure 5.9) (used by permission),
by Christopher Pollitt, BVSc, PhD, DVM,
Associate Professor in Equine Medicine,
School of Veterinary Science,
The University of Queensland,
Qld 4072, Australia.

Clinical Radiology of the Horse, Second Edition,
By Janet A. Butle, Christopher M. Colles, BvetMed, PhD,
MRCVS, Sue J. Dyson, MA, VetMB, PhD, MRCVS,
Svend E. Kold, DVM, DR Med Vet,MRCVS,
Paul W. Poulos Jr, DVM, PhD,
Blackwell Publishing Company, 2000.

Corrective Farriery, A Textbook of Remedial Horseshoeing,
Volume 1,
by Simon Curtis, FWCF, HonAssocRCVS,
R & W Publications (Newmarket) Ltd,
Suffolk, UK, 2002.

Explaining Laminitis and its Prevention,
by Robert A. Eustace, BVSc, Cert EO, Cert EP, FRCVS,
J.W. Arrowsmith Ltd, Bristol, Great Britain, 1992.

Equine Laminitis,
by Christopher C. Pollitt, BVSc, PhD,
RIRDC Publications, Barton, Australia, 2001.

Factors Involved in the Prognosis of Equine Laminitis in the UK,
by R.A. Eustace, BVSc, Cert EO, Cert EP, FRCVS and
P.J. Cripps, BVSc, Bsc, Msc, PhD, MRCVS,
Equine Veterinary Journal, 31.5, 1999.

Farrier Focus Study Guide,
by Doug Butler, PhD, CJF, FWCF,
Doug Butler Enterprises, Inc, LaPorte, Colorado, 2000.

Founder Data Collection and Analysis Form ©,
by Esco Buff, PhD, CF,
Esco Buff's Farrier and Founder Service, Webster, NY, 1990.
www.escobuff.com

Founder Distance Chart (figure 4.2) (used by permission),
by Robert A. Eustace, BVSc, Cert EO, Cert EP, FRCVS,
The Laminitis Clinic, Mead House,
Dauntsey, Chippenham, Wilts SN15 4JA
e-mail - rae@equilife.co.uk

Heart Bar Shoe Update,
by Fran Jurga,
Hoof Care and Lameness, Issue 76, page 41.

Hoof Capsule Rotation Example
(figure 4.1) (used by permission),
by Robert A. Eustace, BVSc, Cert EO, Cert EP, FRCVS,
The Laminitis Clinic, Mead House,
Dauntsey, Chippenham, Wilts SN15 4JA
e-mail - rae@equilife.co.uk

Horse Foot Studies (video),
by Christopher C. Pollitt, BVSc, PhD,
University of Queensland, Australia, 1993.

How to Medically and Mechanically Treat Founder (Video),
by Doug Butler, PhD, CJF, FWCF and George Platt, DVM,
Doug Butler Enterprises, Inc, LaPorte, Colorado, 2001.

Increase Your Chances of Successful Mechanical Treatment For Life-Threatening Founder,
by Doug Butler, PhD, CJF, FWCF,
American Farriers Journal,
September/October, pages 72-8, 2001.

Limb Length Disparity Horseshoeing,
Lecture Handout, Foot Notes - A Clinic For Farriers and Veterinarians, Footlight Farm, Roosevelt, NJ,
by Esco Buff, PhD, CF, 2003.

Limb Length Disparity.
Lecture Handout, Seventh Annual Luwex® Hoof Symposium, Bavaria, Germany,
by Esco Buff, PhD, CF, 2004.

Organizing and Recording Your Founder Cases,
American Farriers Journal,
January/February, pages 105-07, 2003.

The Lame Horse, Causes, Symptoms and Treatments,
by James R. Rooney, DVM,
Wilshire Books Company, 1977.

PBM (Proper Balance Movement), A Diary of Lameness,
by Anthony Z. Gonzales,
REF Publishing, Manassas, Virginia, 1986.

PBM (Proper Balance Movement), Part I,
Confirmation and Lameness (Video),
by Tony Gonzales
Lawlor Productions, San Diego, California.

The Principles of Horseshoeing (P3),
by Doug Butler, PhD, CJF, FWCF and Jacob Butler, CJF,
Doug Butler Enterprises, Inc, LaPorte, Colorado, 2004

Radiological Measurements From the Feet of Normal Horse, With Relevance to Laminitis,
by P.J. Cripps, BVSc, Bsc, Msc, PhD, MRCVS and
R.A. Eustace, BVSc, Cert EO, Cert EP, FRCVS,
Equine Veterinary Journal, 31.5, 1999.

The Importance of Product Freshness,
by Life Data Labs, Inc ®,
Cherokee, Alabama, 2003.

The Veterinary Clinics of North America, Equine Practice, Laminitis,
by David M. Hood, DVM, PhD and
A. Simon Turner, BVSc, MS, DACVS,
W.B. Saunders Company, Philadelphia, PA, 1999.

Proceedings of the Thirteenth Annual AAEP Convention,
Burney Chapman, CJF and George Platt, DVM,
Dallas, Texas, 1984.

Twenty Five Most Frequently Asked Questions About Laminitis,
Special Management Report #8,
American Farriers Journal, 1997.

Vettec Educational Step-By-Step Hand Book, Page 35, Figures 1 and 4, (used by permission),
Oxnard, CA, 2004/2005.
www.vettec.com,

Testimonials From Horse Owners, Farriers and Veterinarians

"Managing a foundered horse has been a nightmare emotionally and financially for the horse owner. The treatment and the prognosis for the founder have been a subjective matter for the Farrier and Veterinarian.

The Veterinarian and Farrier based their decisions on non-tangible signs such as the horse's demeanor, its attitude and their level of experience in the treatment of foundered horses. The owner was left at the mercy of the Farrier and Veterinarian's "best guess" as to their horse's progress.

Esco Buff has presented the horse owner, Veterinarian and Farrier with a very specific methodology for determining the severity of the founder, and more importantly, a methodology for determining progress.

Through a series of specific measurements the horse owner, Veterinarian and Farrier can make an intelligent factual decision on the treatment of the foundered horse and its chances for recovery."
Bob Smith, CF,
Owner of Pacific Coast Horseshoeing School,
Sacramento, California

"To All Horse Lovers,

I may not be the most knowledgeable person when it comes to horses (unlike Esco), but I do love them! In 2001 we had quite a time with our horse, Leo, a sweet paint quarter horse....

We purchased Leo in July, and in August we took a terrible fall. Leo seemed stiff a week or so later, and the barn Veterinarian diagnosed arthritis, and prescribed stall rest and Joint Supplements. Leo was also a bit overweight at the time. We kept him in his stall, and tried to walk him on a lead for a little exercise a few times each week. Needless to say, Leo gained more weight. We had the Veterinarian check his progress again as Leo just never seemed to recover. In addition, Leo started to develop vices like biting. The Veterinarian prescribed bute for the discomfort.

After 3 months we called a new Veterinarian in because Leo was no better. We walked Leo out of his stall and the Veterinarian stopped us almost immediately, telling us, "The horse has very sore feet." Following a series or radiographs and lab test, the Veterinarian diagnosed founder and recommended we call in Esco Buff as the Farrier.
Esco was so wonderful. First he educated us in proper hoof care, diet, and stall conditions for Leo, and then he gave us tons of literature to help us understand founder.

We were shocked to learn that Leo was in a great deal of pain with every step. Just standing caused him terrible

pain. It was no longer a mystery why Leo was off. We were so upset, thinking that our stupidity caused Leo to be worse, but Esco pointed out that others had also missed the diagnosis up to now. Due to the length of time of not being treated, more damage to the foot had occurred.

Esco had to trim Leo's feet, and then fit him with heart bar shoes that would help to relieve some of the pain. The Veterinarian suggested bute, but changed his mind after talking with Esco about the ill effects of foundered horses on bute.

I have never seen anyone like Esco who seems to understand what the horses want, think and feel. He communicates with them in a gentle and compassionate manner, and it's quite wonderful to see. Our horse responds to him so well.

Esco followed up with us via e-mail to inquire how Leo was doing, and kept a regular schedule of treatment. Just as he predicted, we
were riding a sound Leo a year later.

Once again, Leo is pain free, thanks entirely to Dr. Esco Buff. I think I see Leo smile when he sees Esco coming…I know we do."
Jeanne Phillips,
Chronic Type I Foundered Horse Owner,
Canandaigua, New York

"Finally, a clear, concise and easy to use set of directions to evaluate the onset of founder, the progression of individual cases, and a precise language that allows Veterinarians, Farriers and owners to communicate accurately regarding particular cases. These forms have allowed Farriers and I to objectively discuss treatment plans and prognosis in regards to this devastating condition."

Rachel Shuster, DVM
Bordentown, New Jersey

"I honestly believe that if I hadn't found Esco Buff when I did, my horse, Blue would not be here with me now. I only wish I had found Esco sooner so we could have prevented the founder from getting as bad as it was."

Linda Schreiver,
Sinker Horse Owner,
Webster, New York

"I want to let you know how much I learned from your recent clinic on the foundered horse. You relayed a great amount of information. I felt you have good social skills which added to the experience, you interact well with the crowd and made the clinic enjoyable!"

Tony Blackwell, Farrier,
Rainsville, Alabama

"I wish to write this testimonial to extol the virtues of Dr. Esco Buff.

I made his acquaintance after a major stallion at my farm was experiencing founder. The Veterinarians were very concerned about the radiographs and told us to get the best Farrier to help us, a "Master Farrier."

After one very professional visit from Esco, the Veterinarians were tremendously impressed with the improvement in the horse's feet. Even more importantly for me, the horse absolutely trusted Esco. Esco made sure to take the time to make sure that was so.

My stallion was treated with heart bar shoes and in just 6 months was back to being bare footed. To this day, the horse is sound and completely recovered.

Esco is an articulate, knowledgeable and professional Farrier who arrives on time and has a very humane demeanor."
James Maroney, Ennistymon Farm,
Sinker Horse Owner,
Oswego, New York

"Using the Founder Forms on the laminitic or foundered horse enables the Veterinarian and Farrier to more accurately assess and document what is occurring in a horse's foot. This allows for more useful information when determining treatment and prognosis, as well as monitoring a horse's progress."
Jennifer A. Reetz, DVM, DACVIM,
Ontario, New York

"When our horse foundered, it was so bad that our Veterinarian recommended we put our horse, Amanda, down. When we said, "we at least wanted to try and save Amanda," our Veterinarian said "to call Esco Buff."

Not only did Esco save Amanda's life, Amanda was sound and able to be ridden after only one year."
Craig and Cindy Schwartz,
Chronic Type I Foundered Horse Owner,
Marion, New York

"How does your horse feel about your Farrier?

I have come to realize that horses are much smarter than we are, and they know people better than we do. I had my share of incompetent Farriers with my wonderful gelding that foundered because of a thyroid condition. I was unlucky enough to lose my beloved equine friend.

I wish I had Esco Buff as my Farrier during the time my gelding was being treated for founder - an insidious disease that few Farriers know much about, even though they profess to.

Luckily for my mare I found Esco through a good friend. Esco has been my mare's Farrier for a number of years now, and she loves him. She was founder prone with a heavy crest, overweight and also suffering from a thyroid condition. When the dosage was changed, my horse foundered.

I thank my lucky stars that Esco was here. He gave us the options and decided on heart bar shoes immediately. The shoes went on and her relief was immediate.

What a change from what I had been through with my other horse. Her prognosis is good and it is all because of Esco Buff and the heart bar shoe. Not only does Esco consider the comfort of the animal first, he knows what he is doing and teaches you at the same time.

In a world where people act superior with knowledge, here is a man who really has the knowledge and the skill and shares that knowledge and teaches others without hesitation.

And how does your horse feel about your Farrier?

One day when Esco arrived as I was cleaning my mare's stall, I told her "Esco is here, you better get ready." She immediately walked over on the mats in the isle and waited for him. As I finished the stall he did his work on her as she stood there without a bridle or being cross-tied. That's how my horse feels about her Farrier! I'm one of the lucky ones to have Esco as my Farrier."

Marilyn Aldrich,
Limb Disparity Foundered Horse Owner,
Chronic Type I (left fore) and
Chronic Type II (right fore),
Mendon, New York

"We first met Esco in August 2001 when he was called by our Veterinarian to consult on radiographs taken of our horse who had foundered secondary to a viral infection.

Esco took the time to thoroughly examine the radiographs, take measurements, etc. and provide us with the different options available to us in the treatment of our horse. His knowledge of laminitis and founder were extensive and he gave us an honest assessment of our horse's condition and potential final outcome. Given this information, we wanted to proceed.

Knowing that time was of the essence if we were to save this horse, Esco cleared his schedule and spent the entire evening precisely forming and applying heart bar shoes on all four feet of my horse.

Esco encouraged us to educate ourselves as much as we could on the treatment of foundered horses, providing us with the names of books that would give us a wealth of correct information on the subject.

He was familiar with all the different treatments and shoeing methods that are advocated for the treatment of founder and the advantages and pitfalls of them all. Having researched these methods and the statistics on the final outcomes, Esco firmly believes in the use of the heart bar shoes and based on the radiographs, knows how to precisely set them.

Esco encouraged us to ask any and all questions at our initial meeting and further encourages us to contact him with any other questions that arose as time went on (and there were plenty!).

Esco laid out an extensive treatment plan that we should follow to optimize our horse's chances of recovery. He offered encouragement and support as we worked through the initial shock of having something so catastrophic happen to our horse. He remained involved in our horse's care, requiring weekly updates on his condition and answering any further questions we had. He relayed all treatment information to our Veterinarian promptly, advocating a team approach to our horse's treatment.

We are 3 months into the healing process and Esco has been there every step of the way, trimming our horse's feet and resetting his shoes on a regular basis, answering questions and continuing to monitor our horse.

Follow up radiographs show that the heart bar shoe has worked, as evidenced by no further dropping or rotation. Just as important, our horse's pain relief with the application of the shoes was almost immediate and he has remained comfortable. Progress had been excellent to date.

Having researched information through many sources, I have found that generally there are as many theories on the treatment of founder as there are causes. The prognosis given is often variable, and it seems that many people are unfortunate enough not to have access to excellent equine Veterinary care and a skilled Farrier.

With Esco's extensive knowledge of laminitis and founder and his skill in the use of the heart bar shoes, horse owners in our area are fortunate to have this resource available should their horse founder."

Sue Schoen,
Sinker (front) and Acute (hind) Foundered
Horse Owner,
Macedon, New York

"I have been following the suggested founder materials of information dictated by Dr. Esco Buff.

In regards to founder, my clients have immediately noticed the escalation of my success. By shoeing to the numbers and following the Founder Data Collection And Analysis Forms, I get the necessary information to correctly fit and place the heart bar shoe.

The materials presented in this book, should offer the reader and the equine professional along with the owner, hope and a successful outcome.

It is my opinion that Dr. Esco Buff has real solutions to a complex problem."
King A. Lamadora,
Farrier specializing in
Proper Balance Movement (PBM II),
Daly City, California

"Your Founder Data Collection And Analysis Forms have been a real positive in my Farrier practice for the past year and a half. It has helped organize my record keeping and communication with some Veterinarians."
Tom Riney, CJF,
Farrier specializing in dressage horses,
Hailey, Idaho

"This is a story of thanks........................

My story begins of course, with my beautiful Saddlebred mare, Heart. I had discovered that my horse had foundered in early summer of 2002.

I was devastated to say the least. I had no experience with founder, not to mention recovery of founder.
I was at the beginning of my wild goose chase of many suggestions.

At first, My Veterinarian diagnosed her lameness as a bad nail from a previous Farrier. So we removed the shoes and applied a glue on plastic shoe. Two weeks later, she was still lame. My Veterinarian, after my suggestion and urging, returned to radiograph my horse feet. This is when we discovered that she had foundered!

I was instructed to confine her in a stream of water to remove any heat in her feet, or dig a pond for her to stand in. To confine her in a stream somewhere was just not an option, considering there wasn't any water on our property. To make matters worse, we have the driest soil on earth. It's all sand and rocks (bank run soil). So to dig a pond and expect it to hold water was impossible. Keep in mind; this is a horse with a lot of issues.

The main issue is her confinement issue! Her second one is major anxiety! Heart is the leader of my small herd of horses. She is an outstanding kind animal with people, but has major control and separation issues. To make it even more interesting, she is a very hard keeper and a finicky eater.

So now my husband and I are at the point of digging a pond in the paddock so she can still be near the herd. We used a very strong thick pool liner to hold the water and stall mats on top so she wouldn't tear the liner. I took apart my round pen so we could confine her in this 12' x 12' water stall we had made.

After a few hours in the sun, it got to hot for her, so we built a temporary roof over it. She went into the water stall without a problem what so ever. It seemed at first that it was a relief for her. By morning, she had jumped out of the water stall to join the herd! We found her lying in the sand because she was in so much pain. This was the worst thing she could have done for her feet.

Now my Veterinarian suggest that I tranquilize her so she will stay in the stall, and to bute her for the pain. Bute is a big NO-NO with foundered horses (I didn't know this at that time). My Veterinarian did give me one piece of good advise. That was to find a new Farrier who shod foundered horses. I had already decided that on my own already.

As the days rolled on, my horse got worse. Several people had said I should put her to sleep. I was beginning to wonder if that would be the fair thing to do for my friend. I was absolutely beside myself!

After spending a few days on the computer, and my face in several magazines, I came across one little ad for videotape on shoeing foundered horses by Dr. Doug Butler. He is a Certified Journeyman Farrier, teacher, author, publisher and speaker on hoof care. I called the 1-800-728-3826 telephone number right away to order the videotape.

Carla Repke answered the call and she was great! Carla had told me that the first thing I need to do is find a good certified Farrier that could do this procedure that Dr. Doug Butler talks about. I had already been looking for a new Farrier, but hadn't found anyone that would take on this problem.

Carla recommended Esco Buff and said that he had attended Doug Butler's seminars for several years and was using this method to shoe foundered horses.

I called Esco and left a desperate massage. He called back almost right away. I explained everything I could to him and told him about my horse, and what I had been told to do for her. Esco took the time to educate me a little about getting a horse to recover from founder. Everything he said to me made complete sense. He seemed very kind and well educated. I was anxious to meet with him and have him evaluate my horse. I am so glad I did!

I had traveled over six hours with my horse to the clinic that Esco works out of. At the first visit, radiographs were taken; Esco looked over my horse, and then put her in a stall to rest. He spent the next half an hour educating me on the procedure he was about to do on my horse. Then he got busy making measurement from the radiographs and went to work making special shoes for her.

My horse was very relaxed and at ease with him. Esco has a very calm way about him that horses seem to be comfortable with. He is very soft spoken and confident, that is welcoming. Believe me, I've had my fair share of cocky and uneducated Farriers. Esco is just the opposite of that. He was very concerned about getting my horse and myself more comfortable, and he did just that. I had never seen a horse trimmed and shod in this way before.

Just in the first visit, my horse was much more comfortable. My horse has been visiting with Esco on a regular basis since then. It is now the beginning of March 2003, less than a year since my meeting with Esco, and my horse is completely sound again! She now has a regular shoe on and I am working her again. She is a much happier horse at this point and I am so glad I didn't put her down. That would have been a crime.

All I can say is Thank you for all you have done for both of us. Thank you for the hospitality of you and your wife, Christine, for letting me bunk at your house during the harsh winter months, instead of my trailer. The best thing I have to say is I have a new title for you now! You are truly what I call, " The Hoof Whisperer!"
Kimberly Doebel,
Limb Disparity Foundered Horse Owner,
Sinker (left fore) and Acute (right fore),
Accord, New York

"Saying good-bye is always difficult but in this instance it is especially heart wrenching.

You were both "Smoothie" and our savior. Our horse's athletic career has been extended and made possible thanks to your efforts and expertise.

We will feel that we have made a new friend more than a professional acquaintance. Please accept our gratitude and thanks for restoring our noble steed to his former glory."
Mike and Barbara Krefsky,
Severe Limb Disparity Horse Owner,
Robbinsville, New Jersey

"I just wanted to say thanks one more time for all you've done.

After nearly 19 years of owning a horse, I finally met another person with such integrity, empathy and a gift for understanding horses and horse people in general.

Not only did you do wonders for Raajah, but you were very helpful to me during one of the worst days of my life…even though I only knew you one short year, you've been or rather have had a great impact on my life.

You're an incredible person - don't ever change - your children have a wonderful role model. I wish you great things."

Lorrie Scalia,
Limb Disparity Foundered Horse Owner,
Chronic Type I (left fore) and Sinker (right fore),
Marlton, New Jersey

"How do you turn a devastating situation into a better one? The answer is take a beloved equine champion, factor in foundered, then bring in a person at the top of their field. That is what happened to my much loved show mare Hustle To The Limit, aka - Emmy.

In June of 2002, our Veterinarian had us walk and soak her feet for almost two weeks. Our Veterinarian was called out again to re-examine my mare because she steadily had become increasingly lame over the two week time period.

The Veterinarian and our "then" Farrier, both felt that it was an abscess and with that, continued to pare at the sole of her feet. After not finding an abscess during this time, x-rays where finally taken.

I will never forget that afternoon when my mom, after speaking with the Veterinarian, told me the devastating news that Emmy had foundered. It was a blow and a shock to us that was beyond belief.

When you say the work "Founder," everything that I learned in my years of owning and showing equines and even through my years at college for equines, meant that, "if" the horse lived they would be crippled or worthless.

This is so far from the truth when you have Esco Buff in your barn, working with a horse that is willing and able to fight for what could very well be her life.

Esco arrived mid-evening in June to work with Emmy and to also work with us. He explained everything that had happened to Emmy, through the use of her x-rays and his own created Farrier data forms. He pulled books upon books from his trailers bookshelf, in order to give us visuals and knowledge. Esco explained that by looking at Emmy's feet and radiographs, he could tell that she had been foundering for the last five to six months.

I learned that Esco shoes about 60 new foundered cases a year and by taking certain measurements from the x-rays, can give the horse owner a fairly accurate prognosis of survival and use.

Esco gave Emmy a 98% chance of survival and about a 50 % chance of returning to her original soundness state. Esco then went on to explain the work that what would need to be done. And work he did. Esco supported Emmy through heart bar shoes and at some moments, held all of her 16 hands worth of weight on his shoulders just to make it easier on her.

It's been a long way from that June in 2002 to the present (2004). Months of care and corrective shoeing by Esco has brought my mare from what our Veterinarian referred to as a "guarded" condition, to what you see today, a mare on a mission. She runs full out across our arena, bucking, kicking and even gives a little something extra to Esco when he tosses a snowball at her as she plays. As it stands, Emmy and
I will be pairing up to ride again this spring due to Esco.

Esco has given my family so many important things, knowledge, compassion, understanding, friendship and most of all, my horse's life back. He is truly a gift to know, not only professionally, but also personally. We would like to publicly thank Esco from the bottom of all our hearts.

As my mom would like to point out, Esco's business card could not describe him and his business any better; "Providing service that is dependable, caring, ethical and professional." How right she is.
Alice and Cindy Reed
Limb Disparity Foundered Horse Owner,
Chronic Type II (left fore) and sinker (right fore),
Wolcott, New York

"The seminar I attended that was given by Esco Buff, was the most in-depth training in a seminar devoted to the understanding of founder. Esco provides self-instructional detailed learning about Founder, which every Farrier needs to know.

Esco is Highly respected. His experienced methods and clinically proven documentation derived from his detailed data forms, offers the Farrier the opportunity to help diagnose the degree of founder and treat this condition.

As a professional Farrier, I'm highly excited to recommend Dr. Esco Buff's new founder book."
Dwayne Crossland, Farrier,
Delhi, California

"If we wonder often, the gift of knowledge will come." (Arapaho proverb)"

In October, 2003, I attended two clinics in California that featured clinician Esco Buff, PhD, CF.
Esco's experience working with many respected members of our industry on laminitis/founder cases has resulted in a plethora of knowledge, which he enthusiastically passes onto others.

There is a staggering need for correct information to be conveyed to both the Farrier and Veterinary communities. Esco stresses the importance of a good Veterinarian/Farrier relationship.

The goal is a successful return to the horse's state of useful soundness and comfort. The heart bar shoe has been proven to have the greatest success. The problem is, there are more wrong ways than right ways to apply the heart bar shoe. It must be constructed, fit and applied with accuracy.

The clinics proved to be well worth the effort and time to attend. As a Farrier, we depend on our tools for making a living. Upgrading them is a natural progression as our skills improve. Remember, the most important tool is you. Education is an investment in ourselves. No two individuals carry the same combination of talents or challenges. We all have something to gain from the wisdom and experiences of others.

Thank you Esco and all those who hosted the clinics."

"To look at something as though we had never seen it before requires great courage." (Henri Matisse)
Lidia Ivanovna Sawortotnow, Farrier,
Salinas, California

"If you're a horse person, one of the worst things you can hear from your Veterinarian are the words, "it's founder." The day I heard them, I was called to the barn for what I thought was going to be a sprain or muscle strain in my 15-year-old Morgan, Flash. What I encountered was my Veterinarian on the stall floor feeling my horse's pulses. His first words to me were "I'm sorry Fern, Flash has foundered." From that moment, nothing in my life was ever going to be the same again.

The first few weeks were the hardest because I knew a lot less about founder than I thought. I was scared. Things were happening too fast and I was getting more conflicting opinions and advice than I could handle.

As I recall those terrible days, I unfortunately did more panic driven and detrimental things than were wise. Sorting through the advice was the hardest task because I was always sure of one thing - saving my beloved companion from incurring more pain and suffering. I was not prepared for the mental and emotional pain and suffering I too would have to endure.

The next year and a half proved to be a roller coaster of rough and rougher moments. In that time, Flash foundered three more times, abscessed in both feet simultaneously, rotated more and dropped 100 pounds.

People I knew chastised and abused me verbally for seeking solutions and not opting for euthanasia.

My Veterinarian of 10 years "threw in the towel" and told me to prepare for my horse to die, as there was nothing left that he could do. Translation: there was nothing else he knew how to do.

When the entire lateral wall of the right front hoof fell off with a brand new shoe attached, my Farrier of 20 years refused to return because my horse's condition was too poor. Translation: he did not have a clue what he was doing much less what he could do for my horse.

And so, the first month in a brand new barn 26 miles from my home I found myself with a foundered horse with no right foot, no Farrier and no Veterinarian. That was a gift!

Once I recovered from the shock of it all, my mind opened and the solutions dropped in front of me.

First, I became educated in and utilized every feasible treatment complimentary medicine had to offer. I employed several Veterinarians who were amenable to integrative care including Homeopathy, Chinese Medicine, Acupuncture, Chiropractic, Cranial Sacral Therapy, Lymphatic Drainage Therapy, REIKI, and Jin Shin Jyutsu.

Second and most important, I found the right Farrier (thanks to Marilyn Aldrich), who is an expert in the hoof care of foundered horses. Without this kind and compassionate expert, our story would have ended much differently.

There is no one person I can think of who has had a more intense and positive impact on the survival and well being of my horse than Esco Buff. Through every moment of stress and fear, Esco has proven his dedication, knowledge and professionalism and enduring friendship to me. To Flash he has proven his compassion and kindness.

Throughout the last few years, many people have called me about their foundered horses, as I once called others about mine. My advice is simple.

1. Learn everything you can about laminitis/founder and never make a hasty decision because everyone else thinks it's right, because it's the conventional treatment or you are feeling pressured. When in doubt, wait and think about the decision until after you get more information.

2. Educate yourself about what's available, what each treatment is and which practitioners are available to you. Do not be dissuaded by others lack of knowledge. There is no reason why any competent and confident Veterinarian or Farrier should be intimidated or insulted by legitimate use of well orchestrated integrative care.

3. Find the right Farrier. That means someone who is AFA Certified, will actually look at and understand your horse's radiographs and who has expertise in the area of founder. Ask them if they will work with your Veterinarian. If they refuse, keep looking. If

you're lucky enough to live in the surrounding Rochester, New York area, don't walk, RUN to the telephone and call Esco.

4. Take care of yourself because this is a long hard journey, not for the weak or faint of heart. Call people who have lived through the battle of surviving founder. Develop a support system and be willing to offer the same to others when they need you.

5. Offer your horse all the tenderness and comfort you can afford. That may mean some sacrifices on your part. Remember, this is not their fault. You chose this majestic and faithful companion when they were well; they didn't get to choose you. Think about what it would be like to have this happen to you. What would you want done?

6. Expect the unexpected, as it will occur.

7. When others offer their opinion, remember it's theirs, not necessarily yours. Never allow anyone to chastise you for giving good care. Always have faith in what your horse is telling you. Your horse is the best and most truthful source of what is right to do.

8. Don't give up until you are sure there are no more options.

I was fortunate to be befriended by a beautiful, gentle, but very strong and courageous Morgan horse named Lynnmor News Flash. He came into my life when he was 4 years old and gave me unquestionable love and dedication of spirit.

His tragedy at age 15 years old came about through human error - mine. His fate could have been different. Now 7 years later after that horrible day, Flash is still alive, medically healthy and comfortable.

For that gift, we both owe a great deal of gratitude to Esco Buff and the heart bar shoe. Thank you."

"Nyah weh DaNaHo Swenio."

Rev. Fern Hilsinger, BSN, NST, RN,
Chronic Type II Foundered Horse Owner,
Rochester, New York.

"I have taken notice of Dr. Esco Buff for three years, through the Farrier Focus, presented by Dr. Doug Butler.

I had the opportunity to have Dr. Buff give a clinic at the Farrier Center, in Salinas, California. His associate, King Lamadora, followed every detail in the Founder Data Collection and Analysis Form. They shod two chronic cases. In both instances, immediate relief was given to the sore feet. The radiographs and the proper fit and placement of the heart bar shoe made all the difference when treating this disease.

All those who attended the clinic, left well informed and inspired. I want to thank Dr. Esco Buff for his time and his talent."
Michael DeLeonardo, CJF, Farrier,
The Farrier Center,
Harry Patton Horseshoeing Supply,
Salinas, California

To obtain additional copies of this book
or
for more information
contact:

Esco Buff, PhD, CF

At

Esco Buff's Farrier and Founder Service
1347 Robin Hood Lane
Webster, New York 14580

www.escobuff.com

(585) 298-6619